1

Introduction

Introduction

This book is designed for people who need to follow a gluten-free lifestyle because of Celiac disease, gluten sensitivity or gluten intolerance. I prefer to label it a gluten-free "lifestyle" rather than a gluten-free "diet" because that's exactly what it is. A lifestyle – something you must do for the rest of your life. A "diet" is something you follow in order to reach a goal – lose weight, become healthier, etc. Once you reach your particular goal, you can stop your "diet". However, Celiacs must continue their new "lifestyle" – eating gluten-free – for the rest of their lives. There is no end to eating gluten-free. Our goal is to stop being sick and to stay healthy. This is a daily goal, so eating gluten-free must be strictly followed on a daily basis.

If you tell someone you are on a gluten-free diet, the word "diet" brings to mind an image of something you're doing to lose weight. Yes, there are people who eat gluten-free believing it will cause them to lose weight. They do not need to avoid gluten because of health reasons. To them, eating gluten-free IS a diet. Something they can stop whenever they want to. We can't eat gluten if we want to stay healthy. Ever.

If you tell someone you are following a gluten-free lifestyle, the word "lifestyle" brings to mind an image of something you chose to do for the rest of your life. Eating gluten-free IS a lifestyle choice. The alternative is to continue to eat gluten and to continue to be sick. For me, it was an easy choice. I wanted to stop being sick.

The first one in our family to be diagnosed with Celiac disease was my youngest granddaughter. She was 14-months old at the time. Our initial reaction to her diagnosis was, "Oh my goodness – what do we feed her?" The doctor told us we had to feed her food without gluten. We were told gluten was in wheat, rye and barley. Ok, that sounded easy enough. We just stop feeding her foods

1

with wheat, rye or barley in the ingredients, right? We decided to find foods without wheat, since we didn't think we were feeding her many foods with rye or barley. Until you need to read ingredient lists to avoid wheat, you have no idea how many foods contain wheat! And barley, barley malt and rye!

We discovered that manufacturers don't always use the word "wheat" when a product contains wheat. There are other words such as dextrin, semolina, malt, triticale, modified food starch and triticum aestrium to name a few. We researched all the other words that could possibly mean wheat. Holy cow! We were amazed at how many products we were feeding her that actually contained wheat. Not to mention rye and barley.

Much of our learning was by trial and error. I researched Celiac disease and gluten on the internet, but there was SO much information. And much of it was conflicting information. One website would tell me she could eat oatmeal and another would tell me she couldn't. There were differing views on whether or not "just a little gluten" would hurt her or not. It was so confusing and frustrating! Each time she ate gluten she would get so sick – liquid diarrhea, painful abdominal cramps, projectile vomiting, diaper rash that would bleed, and hours and hours of screaming. And each time she ate something with gluten in it and had a reaction, we all felt so guilty. As if we had done this to her on purpose.

Since Aivah's diagnosis, I have been diagnosed with Celiac disease and so have 3 of Aivah's siblings.

We know how confusing it can be when you're told you need to change to a gluten-free lifestyle, but not given much information on HOW to do that. This book is designed to help you live a healthy, nutritious gluten-free lifestyle.

WHAT IS CELIAC DISEASE?

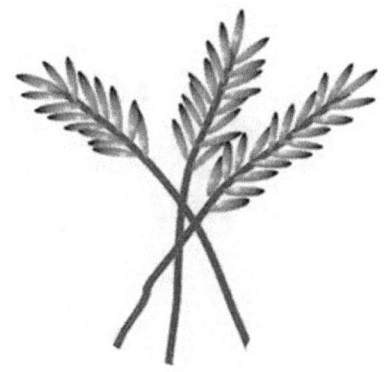

What is Celiac Disease?

Celiac Disease is a permanent, genetic autoimmune disorder that is inherited. It affects 1 in 133 people, however only 3% have been diagnosed. Individuals with Celiac disease cannot digest gluten, a gliadin-like protein that is found in grains such as wheat, rye and barley. There are two classifications of gluten – the prolamines and the glutelins. The prolamine in gluten is called gliadin, which causes the Celiac reactions. The amount of gliadin is what determines the type of reactions a Celiac has. The different levels of reactions are partly due to the amount of prolamines in different grains. The word gluten comes from the Latin word for glue. Gluten gives dough elasticity and strength.

When a Celiac eats gluten, it sets off an autoimmune response that causes inflammation and damage to the villi in the small intestine. Villi are small, finger-like projections that allow nutrients from food to be absorbed through the small intestine and into the bloodstream. Gluten causes the villi to become flattened and unable to absorb nutrients, resulting in malabsorption, meaning nutrients are not being absorbed, and malnutrition. The small intestine is where iron, folic acid, calcium and Vitamins K, A, D and E are absorbed. Celiac disease is also called sprue, Celiac Sprue, non-tropical sprue, Coelic disease (European spelling) and gluten sensitive enteropathy (enteropathy means a disease of the intestinal tract). Celiac disease may be triggered by a stressful situation, such as surgery, severe emotional stress, childbirth or infection. This trigger may cause symptoms to become more pronounced.

Symptoms may vary for each individual depending on their age and the amount of damage that has been done to their small intestine. Because of the wide range of symptoms, Celiac disease can be difficult to diagnose. Many people experience gastrointestinal symptoms such as diarrhea, constipation and flatulence (gas). Others may experience nausea and vomiting (at times projectile vomiting), painful and swollen joints or migraines. In children, failure to grow and thrive can be a signal of undiagnosed Celiac disease. Some individuals do not experience any outward symptoms and are considered "silent Celiacs", yet are still experiencing damage to their small intestine each time they eat food that contains gluten. Celiac disease symptoms can mirror the symptoms of many other health issues, and can make it difficult to diagnose. Studies have shown that if an individual with Celiac disease continues to eat gluten, they have a 40 to 100 times higher chance of developing intestinal or colon cancer.

There is no cure for Celiac disease. You will always have Celiac disease and it will never go away. The only treatment is to follow a strict gluten-free lifestyle. Your symptoms will go away and you will become healthier as long as you follow a gluten-free diet.

If left untreated (continuing to eat gluten), Celiac disease can cause permanent damage to the small intestine. It can become life-threatening and can lead to other conditions such as:

Osteopenia and Osteoporosis
Weight loss
Internal hemorrhaging
Anemia
Delayed start in menstruation
Lack of dental enamel formation
Arthritis
Fibromyalgia
Intestinal and/or colon cancer

SYMPTOMS OF CELIAC DISEASE

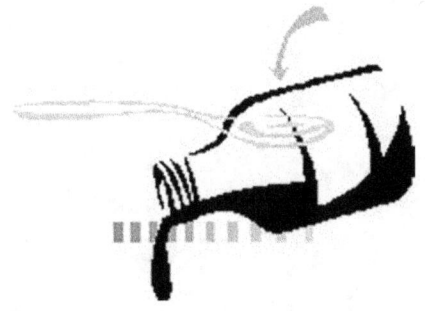

Symptoms of Celiac Disease

The symptoms of Celiac disease result from the inability of the small intestine to digest gluten. Gluten is a protein found in grains such as wheat, rye and barley. Gluten causes damage to the villi of the small intestine. Villi are small, finger-like projections in the small intestines that absorb nutrients as the food passes through. Gluten causes damage by irritating, flattening and shortening the villi. Damaged villi cannot absorb nutrients, resulting in malabsorption of nutrients and malnutrition.

Imagine a truck filled with nutritious food. Normally, the truck stops at every town along his route to leave healthy food for each town. With Celiac disease, the truck "puts the pedal to the metal" and speeds past all the towns, stopping only when it reaches the end of the road. The towns along the route are going hungry and not thriving.

Because of the wide range of symptoms, Celiac disease can be difficult to diagnose. Many people experience gastrointestinal symptoms such as diarrhea, constipation and flatulence (gas). Others may experience nausea and vomiting (at times projectile vomiting), painful and swollen joints or migraines. Some do not experience any outward symptoms and are considered "silent Celiacs", yet are still experiencing damage to their small intestine. Celiac disease symptoms can mirror the symptoms of many other health issues, and can make it difficult to diagnose.

Possible symptoms of Celiac disease can be:

Liquid, foul-smelling diarrhea
Abdominal cramps
Distended abdomen
Headaches / Migraines
Blistered rashes on stomach, buttocks, arms, legs, hands, feet
  (The medical term is Dermatitis Herpetiformis – DH)

Unexplained weight loss
Weight gain
Anemia
High fever
Irritability
Flatulence (gas)
Vomiting (at times projectile vomiting)
Inability to sleep through the night
Bedwetting or incontinence
Listlessness
Low height and weight gain
Dark circles under the eyes
Numerous "cold sores"
Lack of muscle definition
Constipation
Painful, swollen joints
"Brain fog" (the inability to think clearly)

If left untreated, Celiac disease can cause permanent damage to the small intestine. It can become life-threatening and can lead to other health conditions such as:

Osteoporosis
Osteopenia
Bone "pain"
Type 1 Diabetes
Weight loss
Internal hemorrhaging
Central and peripheral nervous system disorders
Anemia
Delayed start in menstruation
ADD / ADHD –type symptoms
Anger issues
Lack of dental enamel formation
Thyroid disease
Liver disease
Rheumatoid arthritis
Hair loss

There is no one specific method of testing and diagnosing Celiac disease. A combination of tests may help with a diagnosis.

Blood Tests

People with Celiac disease have higher than normal levels of certain autoantibodies. These are proteins in their blood that react against their body's own cells. Antibodies are produced by the immune system as a response to a fragment of gluten called gliadin. The antibodies see the gliadin as an intruder and attempt to destroy it. With Celiac disease, the body mistakes its own cells as intruder cells, and destroys healthy cells. The two main areas that can be attacked by antibodies are the covering of the muscle and the framework of the liver and kidney.

These blood tests – sometimes call the Celiac Panel – measure your immune system's response to gluten. This panel tests your levels of anti-endomysium antibodies (EMA) and anti-tissue transglutaminase antibodies (tTGA). You need to be eating gluten before having these blood tests. If you have stopped eating gluten before your blood test, the results may be negative for Celiac disease even if the disease is present. The accuracy of the blood tests is determined by the experience and ability of the pathologist who interprets the results. Test results can vary from one lab to the next, because of a lack of standardization in determining the results. These blood tests are at best, 40-60% accurate and cannot be used alone to determine if a person has Celiac disease. There are many factors that could cause a false-negative result.

Small Intestinal Biopsy

The lining of the small intestine is covered with villi (small finger-like projections.) Celiac disease destroys and flattens the villi, preventing them from absorbing nutrients from the foods we eat. A small intestinal biopsy is currently considered the most accurate test to determine if a person has Celiac disease. A biopsy is an invasive procedure. The patient must be anesthetized while an endoscope is passed through their mouth and stomach into their small intestine. A camera at the end of the endoscope takes pictures of the tissues along the way. Since the damage caused by Celiac disease cannot be seen by the naked eye, it is not possible to confirm a diagnosis just by looking at the intestinal walls. A small instrument is passed through the endoscope and 5-6 tissue samples are taken from the lining of the small intestine. The samples are placed under a microscope and read by a pathologist to determine if the villi have been damaged.

The small intestinal biopsy is currently considered the "gold standard" for diagnosing Celiac disease. Unfortunately, the biopsy is not 100% accurate, either. Celiac disease can cause patchy lesions throughout the small intestine. If the tissue samples are taken from areas that are not damaged, the results will be negative.

DH (Dermatitis Herpetiformis

DH is a skin rash. In intensely itchy, painful skin rash that includes bumps and tiny blisters that contain a clear liquid. Before the bumps and blisters appear, your skin may itch or you may feel a burning on your skin. It normally takes 2-6 days for the bumps to heal. Once the bumps have healed, you may have small, purple marks on your skin from the blisters. These areas may take months to heal. Common areas for this rash are the knees, elbows, buttocks, lower back and the back of the neck, although it can appear anywhere on the body. The gluten circulating in your system causes the skin to react to the gluten antibodies.

DH is diagnosed through a skin biopsy that tests for deposits of antibodies beneath the skin. Medications can be applied to the rash to ease the rash, but the only treatment to "cure" it is to follow a strict gluten-free lifestyle. As long as you continue to eat foods that contain gluten, the rash will remain.

Gluten Elimination Diet

If you have undergone the Celiac panel of blood tests and the intestinal biopsy, but haven't received a positive diagnosis of Celiac disease or gluten sensitivity, you may wish to try a 2-week gluten elimination diet to determine if gluten is causing your symptoms. Neither the blood test nor the intestinal biopsy is 100% accurate.

When you follow a 2-week gluten elimination diet, you eliminate all foods and products that contain gluten for a period of two weeks. During the 2 week period, you may notice an improvement in your symptoms. At the end of 2 weeks, eat a piece of wheat bread. If gluten is causing your body to produce symptoms, the wheat bread will cause your symptoms to return. Your symptoms may come back stronger than before the elimination diet. If gluten is making you sick, your digestive system has had two weeks to begin to heal. Reintroducing gluten may cause diarrhea, nausea, headaches or migraine and brain fog. Since Celiac disease is an autoimmune response, and is NOT a food allergy, it may take up to 48 hours for symptoms to develop. If you don't develop any symptoms after eating wheat bread at the end of the 2-week period, gluten may not be the cause of your symptoms. You should consult your physician to try to determine the cause of your symptoms.

A sample two-week menu, with recipes for many of the gluten-free options can be found at the back of this book.

My daughter had the Celiac panel blood tests run on each of her 7 children. None of the blood tests came back positive for Celiac disease. Two of the tests came back with lower than normal levels, which does not indicate Celiac disease. My daughter and the pediatrician chose not to put all of the children through an intestinal biopsy, since the biopsy is also not 100% accurate. They chose to have each child follow the 2-week gluten elimination diet.

One of the children with a lower than normal blood test had a very bad reaction to eating wheat bread at the end of the elimination diet, that lasted for 3 days. She experienced nausea, diarrhea, migraine, skin rash and brain fog. The other child with a lower than normal blood test experienced nausea, diarrhea and brain fog.

Oddly enough, one of the children with a normal blood test had the most violent reaction to eating the wheat bread. She was sick for 4 days with severe diarrhea, nausea, abdominal cramps, headache, skin rash, lethargy and brain fog.

There isn't just one test that is 100% accurate in diagnosing Celiac disease. Many times, it is a process of elimination. Eliminate what ISN'T causing your symptoms, to discover what IS that is causing them. Symptoms from undiagnosed Celiac disease may range from mild to moderate to severe. My youngest granddaughter, Aivah, experienced many months of painful, frightening episodes before her diagnosis. Her mother tells the story of just one of these frightening experiences.

Words a mommy never wants to hear

I woke up to her whimpering. Not a full cry, just a very slight whimper. I rolled over and felt my little girl, who was sleeping by my side. She was soaking wet, yet burning with fever. This wasn't just any ordinary fever, something was very wrong; I could feel it in my heart. I jumped out of bed, threw on the light and fumbled my way through her drawer. Where was that thermometer???!!!

Underneath one of her many bibs, I found it. I sat on the bed, slowly took her hot, sticky, wet little arm out of her footie jammies. I eased the thermometer under her armpit and heard the beep that it was working. I watched the numbers go up, like I had never seen with my other 6 children. They started so high, 100...102...103...104... Now I was scared, the numbers were still going up. It finally beeped, but I didn't want to look. The fear that took over my body was something I had never felt before. The thermometer read 105.3. I had to look at it 3 times, to make sure I was reading it correctly.

Without even putting her completely back in her jammies, I ran upstairs into my mom's room. I woke her up and told her I had to take Aivah to the hospital, she had a fever of 105.3. She sat up and was immediately aware of what I was saying, not like she usually was if you woke her out of a dead sleep.

I don't even remember the drive to the hospital; it was the longest 15 minutes of my life and every light seemed to turn red, just as I was getting to it. I ran every red light that night. I parked in the spot closest to the door; I didn't even care if it was handicapped or not. I took my baby girl in my arms and ran, as fast as I could, into the Emergency Room. As soon as I told them what her temperature was, they took us back to a pediatric room; nurses and doctors seemed to be swarming us.

They helped me get her out of her jammies and diaper, and asked me to help hold her down. They put an IV into her tiny, little foot; took 3 big tubes of blood from her skinny arm and inserted a catheter. She didn't move, didn't make a single noise, she just held onto my finger with her hot little hand and stared into my eyes.

They put so many medications into that IV, along with the bags of fluids they were trying to hydrate her with. I sat in the rocker, with her in my arms, singing to her while I was saying every prayer I could think of in my head. After an hour, her fever had actually gone up to 105.5 and had no sign of going down, anytime soon.

I thought I felt fear at home, as I sat on my bed staring at that thermometer. When the doctor came in and looked at me, sat on his chair next to mine, held my hand and said, "We can't do anymore here; we need to get her to Minneapolis Children's as fast as we can." That was complete and total fear, words a mommy never wants to hear.

This is how Aivah's story began. We spent many nights at Minneapolis Children's Hospital, many blood tests, stool tests, and high fevers. I should have bought stock in infant's Motrin. The poopy diapers she had were enough to make, even a mommy of 7, gag. The rash she'd get on her little butt was so bad that she would end up with blisters on her tush that would bleed. There were many, many nights spent walking the halls holding a screaming baby. Many nights where all she wanted was to lay in bed, curled up in a ball, crying.

My 13 month old baby girl was only 17 pounds, wore a size 6-9 month clothes and there was absolutely nothing I could do. Thankfully, with the help of a wonderful doctor and a mom that spent all those nights researching, we came across Celiac Disease. The doctor and I decided we should put her on the gluten free diet for two weeks to try it out. Neither of us wanted to put her through an intestinal biopsy because she was so tiny – and the biopsy was only accurate 30%-40% of the time. This would be a true test, he said. We did the diet change and within days she began to turn into a silly, happy little thing with a huge personality.

After the two weeks, we gave her a piece of bread as a 'test'. Within 20 minutes, she was crying, pale, the fever was starting and the diapers were awful again. We told the doctor about the reaction and he told us that, yes, my baby had Celiac Disease.

I was completely overwhelmed with all of the "she'll never..."thoughts. She'll never have a hot lunch at school, she'll never eat one of her friends' birthday treats in class, she'll never have a Happy Meal, she'll never play with play dough... there were so many flying through my head. Then came the grocery shopping – my usual 30 minute trip through the grocery store, turned into 4 hours for the first few months.

During the summer of 2011, we put my other children through the two week elimination diet. It turned out I had 3 more Celiacs!!! All of the "she'll never" thoughts I had in the beginning with Aivah, were now coming true. I now had to figure out how to handle sleepovers with my 13 year old daughter, other children's birthday treats at school with my 10 and 6 year olds, the play dough issue with my 6 year old... Home Economics class with my 13 year old... There are so many things to worry about.

They are all overwhelming, at first. It does get easier and just becomes normal life. The way I have approached it with my kids is that they aren't different, they are just special. If there is a treat at school, I try my best to let the other parents know 'safe' things to bring. If the kids bring cupcakes, if we don't have any on hand, I'll send another treat. When I make meals at home, I can usually alter whatever I'm making for the rest of us so that the 4 of them can have the same thing. Sometimes, I just can't alter something, so they get to choose from one of the alternate meals.

The most confusing part is that I have 2 that are just gluten-free and 2 that are gluten- and dairy-free. I also had to accept the fact that the kids, and even I, will make mistakes sometimes and not realize it until it's already been eaten. We've found that Tums, yogurt (soy yogurt for the dairy free ones), Motrin, Altoids and just plain sleep helps when they've accidentally gotten eaten gluten. The biggest suggestion I have for other new Celiac parents is – teach your kids to be active in their disease. Teach them all the things to look for in food, teach them to ASK QUESTIONS wherever they are, and teach them all of the possible things that 'could' happen later in life if you cheat on your diet. Most of all -- teach EVERYONE in their lives that this is a disease. It is not an allergy. Just because your child won't need immediate medical attention after eating gluten, like they would with a peanut allergy, this is still just as serious.

From one parent of many Celiacs, just relax and remember knowledge is the key to having a healthy, happy child with Celiac Disease.

GLUTEN SENSITIVITY
OR
WHEAT ALLERGY

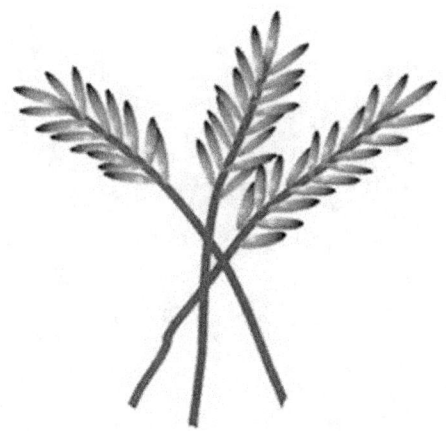

Gluten Sensitivity or Wheat Allergy

Non-Celiac Gluten Sensitivity is more difficult to diagnose. Individuals who suffer from Non-Celiac Gluten Sensitivity experience many of the same symptoms as people with Celiac Disease. However, the blood test which identifies and diagnoses Celiac disease comes back as negative. The only way to diagnose gluten sensitivity is by eating a gluten-free diet for a minimum of two weeks. During this two week period, if you adhere to a strict gluten-free lifestyle, your symptoms should lessen or go away completely. At the end of the two week period, you eat a slice of wheat bread. If you experience the same symptoms as before your gluten-free trial, gluten sensitivity may be the diagnosis. If you do not have a reaction after eating gluten, your symptoms are not being caused by gluten sensitivity, but some other health condition.

Gluten sensitivity, also known as gluten intolerance, is a condition where they body has an immune reaction after eating foods containing gluten. Symptoms of gluten sensitivity are similar to those of Celiac disease. Symptoms can include one or more of the following: liquid, foul smelling diarrhea; headaches; abdominal cramping; unexplained weight loss; vomiting (at times projectile); inability to sleep through the night; listlessness; dark circles under the eyes; constipation and more.

Wheat is one of the top 8 food allergens in the United States that must be stated on food labels. An allergy to wheat is different from Celiac disease or gluten sensitivity and does not involve the immune system. A wheat allergy is a histamine response to wheat, much like a peanut allergy or hay fever. Symptoms of a wheat allergy are not the same for everyone. Some people experience hives while others might experience stomach pain and diarrhea. The most basic negative response is an allergic reaction to wheat that quickly brings on hives, congestion, nausea or potentially fatal anaphylaxis. An allergy is the response of white blood cells called basophils and mast cells to something called Immunoglobulin E (or IgE for short). You develop antibodies to an allergen, in this case wheat. Many individuals with a wheat allergy can tolerate other grains such as rye and barley, since it is specifically wheat that causes an allergic reaction, not gluten (which is also in rye and barley).

It is important to distinguish between Celiac disease, gluten sensitivity and a wheat allergy. Celiac disease is an inherited autoimmune disease that causes permanent damage to the small intestine. Individuals with Celiac disease are at risk for nutritional deficiencies and may develop other autoimmune conditions and cancers. Individuals with a gluten sensitivity/intolerance or a wheat allergy do not usually have severe intestinal damage and are not at risk for nutritional deficiencies. They also do not have an increased risk of developing other autoimmune conditions. Due to the differences between these conditions, and the risk of developing nutritional deficiencies, other autoimmune conditions and cancers, it is important to receive a correct diagnosis.

BRAIN FOG and BODILY FUNCTIONS

Brain Fog and Bodily Functions

Whether I accidentally eat food with gluten in it or "just" get cross-contaminated, the one side effect I really, really don't like is the brain fog. When your thought process works fine – for all of 5 minutes – and then you can't remember what you were doing. I can be having a normal conversation and will lose my train of thought right in the middle of a sentence. Or when words disappear from my head. In the middle of a conversation, I'll forget a common word like "bird". It's like I can look inside my head and know where the word is, but when I try to look at that spot instead of seeing the word I want, I see an empty hole. Eventually, the word reappears but by then I've forgotten why I needed the word in the first place. My brain isn't like this all the time when I get gluten, it comes and goes. I can be "normal" for hours and then the fog rolls in for 20 – 30 minutes and I have to dig my way out of it again.

I remember this was how I felt most of the time before I went gluten-free. Back then, I thought THIS was normal – it was how I felt every day. That was back before I was able to discuss the dreaded "bodily functions" with other people. In public. Since that time, I have discovered if you have Celiac disease, you NEED to learn to discuss bodily functions – like diarrhea, constipation, nausea, belching, burping, gas, abdominal cramping and vomiting. You can't possibly be queasy about discussing bodily functions. It's so much a part of our Celiac life. It doesn't bother me to talk about the various bodily functions any longer. I have a harder time discussing the brain fog. Everyone has bodily functions, some more often than others. Another Celiac will be able to relate to brain fog, but the general public can't. If you've never experienced it, it's hard to imagine what it's like. I'm always worried that when I try to explain what brain fog is, people will just assume I'm trying to find an excuse for memory loss, or they might worry I have the start of Alzheimer's.

I know that I only get brain fog when I've had gluten. I know it will only last a day or two (off and on) when I've been cross-contaminated with a slight amount of gluten. I know it will last 3 – 4 days when I've actually eaten something with gluten in it. I also know that the brain fog isn't the only side-effect I will get from gluten. I know by my symptoms if I've just been cross-contaminated or if I actually ate gluten by the severity of the symptoms. I know this is different for everyone, but I thought I'd share my symptoms. You may be able to say, "Hey, I have that too!"

With a slight gluten contamination (such as eating a chip that has been manufactured in the same plant or on the same lines as gluten foods) the first thing I notice is I hold my breath. When I hold my breath, my abdomen doesn't hurt as much. However, I notice I'm holding my breath BEFORE I notice that I have abdominal pain. The breath holding is sort of a warning sign that the rest of my symptoms will soon follow. It starts with a tightening in my upper abdomen, not really painful. About an hour or two after I notice I've started holding my breath, the abdominal cramps begin. Then the nausea. It sort of comes and goes. I finally understand what a "wave of nausea" is. It will rush over me like a dark, rolling storm cloud. At times It's so strong I feel lightheaded, so sure I'm going to throw up. Slow, deep breaths seem to help. Just about the time I think the nausea is going to succeed, it's gone. It lets me believe it's gone for, oh, at least 15 minutes. Then it rolls in again and I go through it all over again. This process normally lasts for 4 – 6 hours. Mixed in with the nausea is the headache. Not a migraine that makes me seek darkness and complete silence, just a sort of sick, icky headache. A few hours later and I know the gas pains will be upon me. There are times I could swear I was in labor all over again, if I didn't know better. At least, with labor, you get a sweet little baby at the end of it. With gluten contamination, all you get are gas pains that snap you in half and take your breath away until they make their way through. At this end of all this, of course, is the diarrhea. This will all last 24 - 36 hours before it leaves.

However, when I get a larger dose of cross-contamination or actually eat something with gluten IN it (as opposed to ON it), It's an entirely different story. It begins the same, with holding my breath to avoid the abdominal pain. At this point, I don't know if it's from cross-contamination or from actually eating gluten. Within two hours, however, I will definitely know. Instead of an abdominal tightening, it's full speed ahead right into severe abdominal cramps. Someone is inside of me, grabbing handfuls of my intestines, twisting and trying to rip them out. Diarrhea doesn't take its time, either. Slam, bam, let's not leave the house! The one-sided headache slams right into migraine. Pound, pound, pound, pound! If my head were to explode, it wouldn't surprise me. It would probably hurt less than the migraine! Of course, I have nausea. The thought of food just makes it worse. And then nausea slides right into vomiting. (I really, really hate to throw up!) These severe symptoms will last a minimum of three to four days, and then slowly fade away.

I will say, I'm getting much better at pretending I'm ok when I'm not. People tend to get nervous around someone who seems to be sick all the time, regardless of what you tell them is causing it. I'm not sure if they think they can catch what I have or if they just think I'm a hypochondriac. I guess it doesn't really matter.

It also doesn't matter if I know I'll be through the symptoms in 2 days or in 4 days – my "treatment is the same. When I realize I've started holding my breath, I take two Acidophilus. This is a probiotic that helps to balance your "internal flora." I love to use that phrase – it drives my grandkids crazy! They've learned not to ask what "flora" is – because they know I'll go into lecture mode and explain it to them in detail. Internal flora is the microbes and other germs that live in our stomach, small and large intestines and colon. That delicate balance gets out of whack when Celiacs are "glutenized". The Acidophilus puts them back into balance. If you choose to take Acidophilus, be sure to buy the capsules that are kept in the refrigerator section. They contain the live cultures you need. The tablets that are kept on the shelf have been heated in order to compress them into hard, round little tablets. The heating and compressing kills the live cultures.

I wait to see if the diarrhea will start. It always does, but each time I play a game with myself and give myself the false hope that maybe THIS time I won't get diarrhea. But I do. As soon as it starts, I take two slippery elm bark capsules. These capsules contain the inner bark that has been scraped from inside the outer bark of the slippery elm tree. It has been used by Native Americans for many medicinal purposes. It soothes the digestive tract and is a demulcent substance. A demulcent (derived from the Latin word demulcere, meaning "caress") is an agent that forms a soothing film over mucous membranes, relieving pain and inflammation of the membrane – Wikipedia). It will not turn diarrhea into constipation (we don't need that problem). It just "slows things down" and puts it all back to a "normal" consistency. (See? I can discuss bodily functions in detail.) I want to get rid of the gluten in my system, but I want to be as comfortable as I can during this process.

My third step is ginger. I prefer candied ginger, which tends to have a "bite" to it. My grandchildren (four of whom are Celiacs) prefer gluten-free gingersnaps. What's not to like about eating cookies to make you feel better? If you choose gingersnaps, be sure to buy the brand(s) that use real ginger in their cookies. Ginger "flavor" will not help. If I'm out of candied ginger or gingersnaps, I eat Altoids® mints. They use natural peppermint oil in their candies, which also help to relieve the nausea and abdominal cramps.

After this, I just wait it out. There isn't much else you can do but let the gluten work its way through your system and hope it's a fast trip this time.

These are the steps I take when I have been "glutenized". They work for me. They may not work for everyone. It is up to each individual to determine which products are safe for them.

Sometimes we think everyone reacts the same way we do. Or we think no one else has the same reactions and we're in this alone. Neither one is right, but it's nice to know there are other people out there who go through the same things you do. Bodily functions and brain fog are part of being a Celiac. It's what we do. It's what we live with. The key word here is "we". We are not alone.

CROSS-CONTAMINATION

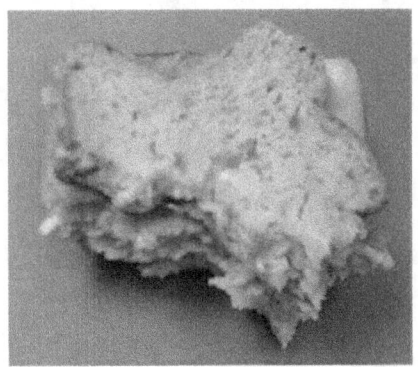

Cross-contamination

Cross-contamination occurs when a gluten-free food comes into contact with a food or a surface than contains gluten. Cross-contamination is a very real problem for individuals who follow a gluten-free lifestyle. There are steps you can take to avoid cross-contaminating your gluten-free food. Gluten is invisible to the naked eye, but can contaminate surfaces such as counters, cutting boards and utensils.

A good example is making two peanut butter sandwiches. One sandwich is made with wheat bread and the other is made with gluten-free bread. You set two pieces of wheat bread on the counter. Then, you spread the margarine and peanut butter on the wheat bread. You cut the sandwich in half and place the halves on a plate. You remove the knife you used, the margarine and the jar of peanut butter you used for the wheat sandwich. Now you are ready to make the gluten-free peanut butter sandwich. You take out the gluten-free margarine, the gluten-free peanut butter, the gluten-free bread and a new knife. You set the gluten-free bread on the counter . . . . . . and you've just contaminated the gluten-free bread with the gluten that is on the counter from the previous wheat sandwich! You can't see the gluten, but it's there on the counter.

If you are going to make toast with gluten-free bread, you will need two separate toasters. Once you place a slice of wheat bread in a toaster, it is contaminated and cannot be used for gluten-free bread. It isn't necessary to purchase separate knives, forks and spoons to be used only for gluten-free foods. You can share utensils between foods that contain and gluten-free food, but they must be washed thoroughly between the two foods. There is no need to purchase a new set of pots, baking pans or dishes to be used specifically for the gluten-free food. However, you do need to pay close attention to how you take care of these pans and dishes. A thorough washing will remove the gluten from them. If you use wooden spoons, it is a good idea to use separate wooden spoons for foods that contain gluten and gluten-free foods as gluten can be absorbed into the wood. Plastic storage containers need to be separated, also. Plastic can absorb gluten (the same way they absorb orders and colors) and may contaminate any gluten-free food you store in it. Be sure to mark the gluten-free plastic containers clearly. Foods that will not be consumed in one serving, such as margarine, peanut butter, mayonnaise, etc. need to be duplicated. One set for those who needs to eat gluten-free foods, another set for those who are able to eat foods that contain gluten. If you use a knife to spread margarine on a piece wheat bread, the knife is contaminated with gluten and cannot be put back into the margarine without contaminating the entire container. Keep the gluten-free food and the food that contains gluten in separate containers. Any food that can be served out of its container, such as peanut butter, mayonnaise, sour cream or margarine, need to be kept in duplicate. You will need two containers of each food. It's too hard to remember not to put your knife or your spoon into the container on foods that contain gluten. The first time someone forgets, and puts their knife into the margarine after touching bread that contains gluten – the entire container of margarine is contaminated.

The same "keep it separate" rule applies to gluten-free flours. Do not store gluten-free flours in the same cupboard as the flours that contain gluten. The possibility of cross-contamination is too high. Store all non-perishable gluten-free foods in a separate cupboard. We also separate gluten-free foods in the refrigerator - they have their own drawer. The chapter on "Your Gluten-free Kitchen" explains this in more detail.

Cross-contamination can be a very big problem when eating in restaurants. A restaurant may advertise that they offer gluten-free foods. However, if they cook their gluten-free foods alongside the foods that contain gluten, you no longer have gluten-free food. It has been contaminated by the foods that contain gluten. If a restaurant uses the same utensils on gluten-free foods and foods that contain gluten, your food is no longer gluten-free. A chef stirs chicken noodle soup with wheat noodles with a metal spoon. He then stirs the gluten-free soup with rice noodles with the same spoon. The gluten-free soup is no longer gluten-free. Many people understand that foods need to be prepared with gluten-free <u>ingredients</u>. Unfortunately, they don't always understand the cross-contamination issues. Always check WHERE the restaurant is cooking their gluten-free foods, and if they use separate cutting boards, pans and utensils. Do they wash their hands before touching any gluten-free food? Do they change their plastic gloves after touching food that contains gluten? Don't be afraid to ask detailed questions about how the gluten-free food is prepared and served. There are many people who are choosing to follow a gluten-free diet in order to lose weight, or because they feel it's healthier for them. They don't need to eliminate gluten from their diet because it makes them sick. Cross-contamination is not going to be an issue for them.

In addition to offering foods that don't contain gluten ingredients, restaurants need to be careful how they prepare their food. They need to train their entire staff on the proper way to handle gluten-free foods and educate them about the dangers of the smallest amount of cross-contamination. If you are not satisfied with the answers you receive at a restaurant you can either offer to educate and train their personnel about gluten or find another restaurant to eat at.

You need to remember that even though a product is listed as gluten-free, it must also be manufactured in a facility that is dedicated only to gluten-free foods to be truly gluten-free. Many manufacturers make products with gluten-free ingredients, but also manufacture products that contain gluten in the same plant. If so, there is a risk of cross-contamination. To be truly gluten-free, a food must be manufactured in a separate area where there is no chance of cross-contamination. Many companies state on their labels that the food is manufactured in the same plant as gluten or wheat products. I am very sensitive to the smallest amount of gluten and have discovered (the hard way) that I need to avoid all products that state they were manufactured in a facility that also manufactures wheat products. Since there are many levels of reactions to gluten, each individual needs to decide for themselves which foods are safe for them to eat.

The best way to find out if a product contains gluten or is manufactured in a gluten-free facility is to call the manufacturer and ask. You may need to talk to more than one person to get to the right department, but it is well worth the effort. It is a good idea to keep a list of these phone numbers on hand. Manufacturers introduce new products and change ingredients in many of their products without notice and you may need to call them more than once to check on their products.

Food isn't the only thing to be concerned with. Products such as toothpaste, lotions, shampoos, band-aids and medicines can also contain dairy or gluten. Some people are sensitive to personal care products that contain gluten and can develop Dermatitis Herpetiformis (DH). DH is an extremely itchy, red rash that is made up of bumps and tiny blisters. The rash can remain on the skin for an extended period of time, before clearing up. Some people are not that sensitive to touching products that contain gluten. The only way to know if your skin will react to touching gluten is trial and error.

READ THE INGREDIENTS before purchasing anything. Believe me, this becomes second nature. Eventually, each time you pick up a product, you automatically turn it around to read the ingredient list before you consider purchasing it.

As always – it is up to those following the gluten-free lifestyle to determine if a product is safe for them.

RECOGNIZING "Gluten" ON INGREDIENT LISTS

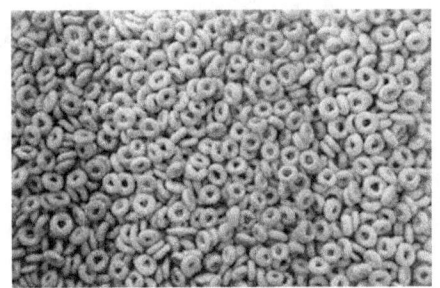

Recognizing "Gluten" on ingredient lists

Shopping for a gluten-free lifestyle can be confusing and frustrating. It's easy to spot "gluten" or "wheat" on an ingredient list. But what of those long, unrecognizable words you find on ingredient lists? Words like Semolina, Triticale or Hydroxypropyltrimonium? Do most people know that those are also words for "gluten"? When I first began grocery shopping after my granddaughter was diagnosed with Celiac disease and a Casein (dairy) allergy, my shopping trips increased from 20 minutes to an hour or more. Since I discovered I also need to eat gluten-free (and dairy-free) I can't imagine buying something without turning it over to read the ingredient list. Anyone with Celiac disease or gluten intolerance has had this same experience.

Not only do you need to look at the actual ingredients on every product, but you also need to look at the type of facility the food was manufactured in. Was it manufactured in a facility that also manufactures products with wheat? If so, there is always the possibility of cross-contamination. I have eaten some gluten-free products that were manufactured in a facility that also manufactures wheat products and had no problem. There are other products that made me very sick. The products themselves contained no gluten, but they had been contaminated in the manufacturing facility. Many companies state that their machinery is cleaned after processing wheat products, before any gluten-free products are processed. Unfortunately, gluten is invisible and if every nook & cranny on the machinery is not cleaned thoroughly, there is always a chance for cross-contamination.

Keep in mind there are many levels of reactions to gluten. Some people cannot tolerate even trace amounts of gluten without getting a physical reaction. Some can eat food manufactured in the same plant with gluten products and feel fine. There are also those individuals who don't experience any outward symptoms yet still have Celiac disease which is causing damage to their intestinal tract.

The US Federal Government has determined that a product with 20ppm (parts per million) can be considered gluten-free. 20 parts per million means 20 milligrams per kilogram of food. Put into language I can understand, that means that 1 kilogram of food (which equals 2 lb 3 oz) can contain 20 milligrams (0.000705 oz) of gluten and still be considered gluten-free. Granted, that isn't much, but for some of us it is still enough to cause a reaction of diarrhea, nausea, migraines, Dermatitis Herpetiformis and brain fog. I speak from experience, here. My experience and the experience of two of my grandchildren. I have two other grandchildren with Celiac disease that don't have a reaction to 20ppm of gluten in their food. Whether you have a reaction or not, is it enough gluten to cause damage to your intestinal tract? I don't know for sure.

OTHER NAMES FOR GLUTEN

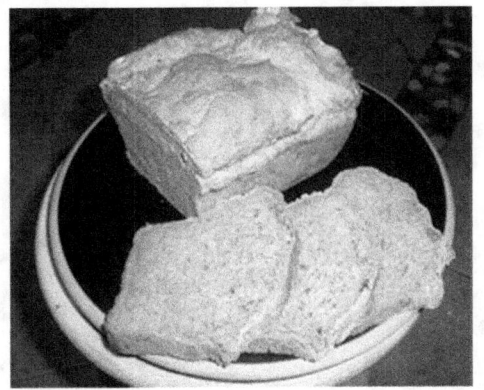

Other Names for Gluten

Gluten can be in items that include wheat or wheat by-products (or rye or barley products), but are not as easily recognized as the word "wheat". Gluten is also in rye, barley, spelt and other grains which are used to manufacture many products. The list below is not an absolute list of ingredients that contain gluten, but the most commonly found on ingredient lists.

Please read your ingredients. If you or your child has a gluten sensitivity or Celiac disease, avoid the following:

Alcohol
Distilled alcohol can be made from grains such as wheat and are not gluten-free. This includes the alcohol used as a base for flavorings such as vanilla used in cooking. Most wines are gluten-free. Most beer is NOT gluten-free (unless it specifically states Gluten-Free Beer). If in doubt, call the manufacturer and ask what the alcohol is made from.

Artificial Colors
The majority of food colors are made from petroleum. They are a derivative of Petrochemicals and Coal tar. Many food colors are pulled off of the market regularly because of health concerns. Yellow #2 food dye has been shown to cause ADHD, multiple types of cancer, male sterility, and many other issues. Yellow 5, Red 40, and six other widely used artificial colorings have been linked to hyperactivity and behavior problems in children.

Many food colors are made from natural ingredients and there are brands that are gluten-free. McCormick and Wilton are two brands that are gluten-free.

Barley
Barley is a cereal grain and <u>does</u> contain gluten.

Bleu Cheese

The "blue" color in Bleu Cheese actually comes from mold. Many manufacturers use wheat bread to "grow" the mold. Some Bleu Cheese is gluten-free, some Bleu Cheese is not - verify by reading ingredients or calling the manufacturer.

Bran

Bran is the hard outer layer of grains such as wheat, barley and rye and is NOT gluten-free. Rice bran IS gluten-free, but must specifically state RICE bran.

Caramel Color

The problem with caramel color is it may or may not contain gluten depending on how and where it is manufactured. The color additive caramel is the dark-brown liquid resulting from heat treatment of the following food-grade carbohydrates: Dextrose (corn sugar), invert sugar, lactose (milk sugar), malt syrup (usually from barley malt), molasses (from sugar cane), starch hydrolysates (can include wheat), sucrose (cane or beet). In the US food, manufacturers use corn to produce caramel color. Caramel color is on the "safe" list for Celiacs, as long as it has been manufactured in the United States.

Couscous

Couscous is a dish made by rolling and shaping moistened semolina wheat and then coating the pieces with finely ground wheat flour. It is NOT gluten-free.

Dextrimaltose

Dextrimaltose is a carbohydrate and is NOT gluten free when it is processed by the enzymatic action of barley malt on corn flour.

Dextrins

Dextrin is a carbohydrate formed by the application of dry heat on starch, such as wheat, corn, potato or rice. If it is produced from wheat, "wheat" will be shown on the ingredient list.. Dextrin added to water forms a sticky gum used as a food thickener.

Durum Semolina
Semolina is derived from the Latin word simila meaning "flour". Durum Semolina is made from durum wheat.

Edible starch, Food Starch (Corn Starch is gluten-free)
The 'starch' could be from corn, wheat, potato, rice or tapioca. Unless it specifically states "Food starch from corn" (or potato or rice or something other than a grain such as wheat or rye) assume it is NOT gluten-free and avoid it.

Food Starch, Modified
Modified food starch is a starch that has been treated physically or chemically to modify one or more of its physical or chemical properties. The 'starch' could be from corn, wheat, potato, rice or tapioca. If wheat was used in the manufacture of the food starch, "wheat" will appear on the label. In the US, if food starch is derived from wheat, manufacturers must state "wheat" on the label as a possible allergen. Wheat is one of the top 8 allergens in the US.

Einkorn
Einkorn wheat is one of the oldest groups of wheat.

Glucose syrup
Glucose syrup is a sugar substitute made from a combination of glucose, dextrose and maltose. It is gluten-free.

Groats
Groats are hulled grains such as wheat and barley.

Hydrolyzed wheat protein
The key word "wheat" tells you this is NOT gluten-free.

Hydrolyzed wheat gluten
The key word "wheat" tells you this is NOT gluten-free.

Hydrolyzed wheat starch
The key word "wheat" tells you this is NOT gluten-free.

Hydroxypropyltrimonium hydrolyzed wheat protein/starch
The key word "wheat" tells you this is NOT gluten-free.

Kamut®
All wheat belongs to the genus Triticum. Kamut® brand wheat is a khorasan wheat.

Malt (flavoring, extract, syrup)
Malt is made by processing grains, usually barley. Malt is NOT gluten-free.

Miso
Miso (fermented bean paste) is a concentrated, savory paste made from soybeans--often mixed with a grain such as rice, barley, or wheat and is NOT considered gluten-free

Modified food starch
Modified starch is prepared by physically, enzymatically, or chemically treating native starch, thereby changing the properties of the starch. If wheat was used in the manufacture of the food starch, "wheat" will appear on the label. In the US, if food starch is derived from wheat, manufacturers must state "wheat" on the label as a possible allergen. Wheat is one of the top 8 allergens in the US.

MSG (monosodium glutamate)
MSG is a commonly used food additive and is considered gluten-free. However, many Celiacs cannot tolerate MSG. (See Chapter on MSG for more information.)

Maltodextrin
Maltodextrin is classified as a sweet polysaccharide. It is usually made from wheat, rice, corn, or potato starch. Maltodextrin is produced by cooking down the starch. During the cooking process, which is often referred to as a hydrolysis of starch, natural enzymes and acids help to break down the starch even further. The end result is a simple white powder. Maltodextrin is such a highly processed ingredient that the protein is removed, rendering it virtually gluten-free

Maltose (malt sugar)

Maltose is also known as malt sugar. Maltose is formed by uniting two units of glucose that provide the first link in a process that results in the creation of starch. When a germinated grain, such as barley, is combined with water and heated the enzymes break down the starch in the grain to produce maltose. Maltose made from wheat, rye or barley is NOT gluten-free.

Oats

You must be sure you are purchasing Certified Gluten-free Oats. Oats themselves do not contain gluten. However, oats are generally cross-contaminated in the fields because of crop rotation, by machinery that is used to harvest both oats and wheat, and in facilities that manufacturing oats and other grains.

Semolina

Semolina is the coarse, purified wheat middlings of durum wheat.

Soy sauce

Regular soy sauce is generally wheat-based. There is GF soy sauce and GF Tamari - but verify it is states that it is gluten-free on the label. There is also a wheat based Tamari.

Smoke flavoring

Smoke flavoring is derived from burning various woods, including hickory and mesquite. Barley malt flour may be used as a carrier for the captured "smoke." Some manufacturers list the sub-ingredients of the smoke flavoring used in their products; others do not.

Spelt

Spelt is a wheat, Triticum aestivum spelta

Starch (see Food Starch)

Tabbouleh
Tabbouleh is a combination of nutty cracked wheat or bulgur mixed with ripe tomatoes, cucumbers, and green onions, mint and parsley.

Teriyaki Sauce
Teriyaki sauce is an oriental sauce used for cooking made with soy sauce and other ingredients. If the ingredient list includes "soy sauce" the soy sauce is generally made from wheat. There are GF soy and teriyaki sauces, but it must state "gluten-free" on the label.

Texturized Vegetable Protein
Most texturized vegetable protein is made from soy protein - and is gluten-free. There are, however, texturized vegetable proteins made from grains that contain gluten. READ THE LABELS.

Triticum Aestrium
Triticum Aestivum is a species of wheat and is NOT gluten-free.

Triticale
Triticale is a hybrid of wheat and rye and is NOT gluten-free.

Vegetable starch
Vegetable starch is generally gluten-free, unless "wheat" is noted on the label

Wheat Germ
Wheat germ is a part of the wheat kernel and is NOT gluten-free.

THE EMOTIONS OF GLUTEN-FREE

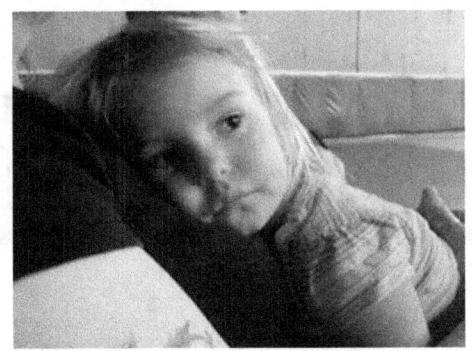

The Emotions Gluten-Free

When you are diagnosed with Celiac Disease or gluten sensitivity there is a myriad of emotions you may experience. These emotions are a normal process to accepting your new lifestyle.

Relief

Once you receive a diagnosis of Celiac disease, your initial reaction is relief. Relief that you finally know WHAT is wrong with you or your child. For many of us, it can take years before finally reaching a diagnosis. On average, it takes most people with Celiac disease 11 years before they are correctly diagnosed. (I was 56 when I was diagnosed and had been to doctors with various symptoms for more than the average 11 years)

You may have experienced symptoms for years. You may have attributed those symptoms to other health issues and accepted them as a normal part of your life. You may have seen numerous doctors. You may have been tested and/or treated for other health issues such as IBS (irritable bowel syndrome), Crohn's disease, blood disease, tumors, cancer, cystic fibrosis or depression. You may have been treated as if you were a hypochondriac or told your child just had "growing pains". Maybe you were told it was "all in your head".

Most of us have been through the symptoms. (Some Celiacs are asymptomatic, so may not have any outward symptoms.) When you do receive a diagnosis, it's finally a relief to know WHAT has been causing your symptoms. It's nice to be able to put a name to the cause of your illness. Not knowing what is causing you to be sick can be frightening. Your mind creates all sorts of scenarios. Sometimes you wonder if there will ever be an end to being sick.

A diagnosis and a name – Celiac disease or gluten sensitivity – is something. It brings some relief to know WHAT it is.

Panic

This relief can be short-lived and slide right into panic. When you are told you need to remove gluten from your diet or your child's diet, and you find out how many foods contain gluten, the next step may be panic. What do I eat? What can I feed my child? At first, it seems as though there is gluten in everything. From food to soap to shampoo to lotion to make-up to toothpaste. Is there anything we CAN eat or CAN use? Does that mean no sweets? Is there any bread we can eat? What about school and family gatherings and birthday parties and eating out? Does this mean we have to avoid going anywhere? It can feel overwhelming at the beginning.

When my granddaughter was first diagnosed, we didn't panic for about a week. It took that long to research wheat and gluten and other names for gluten and Celiac disease in order to have a basic understanding of gluten. It took that long to learn how to read an ingredient list. It took that long to realize they put gluten IN JUST ABOUT EVERYTHING! Believe me, we experienced panic. Don't let yourself be consumed by panic. Take the time to educate yourself. Learn what foods are safe, where to shop for gluten-free foods and what to look for on an ingredient list. Once we found a selection of foods that were safe, the panic began to fade. There are many more companies offering gluten-free foods today than ever before. Believe me, it DOES get easier.

Fear

After panic, is the fear that we will eat the wrong food and become sick, again. We have lived with our symptoms for a long time. Now that we know there is a way to finally be rid of those symptoms and feel healthy, we don't want to go back there again. There is the fear that we will forget to read an ingredient list, or a manufacturer will find a new word to describe wheat or rye or barley and we won't know. We know what the reactions to eating gluten are – we don't want to go through that or put our children through that if we can avoid it. Don't let yourself be consumed with fear to the point where you are afraid to eat or feed your child. Education is the key. Learn about gluten, where it is, what it's called, what foods are safe to eat. Teach your child about Celiac disease – what gluten can do to their body and how it can make them sick if they eat foods that contain gluten. You can't be with them 24 hours a day. They can't always be sure the adults around them understand Celiac disease and cross-contamination. They need to be able to make informed choices about the foods they eat. Teach them how to read an ingredient list (or if they are too young to read, teach them to ask questions. My youngest granddaughter could ask "Is it gluten-free?" when she was 2 ½. And she knew that if her food had gluten in it, she would get sick.) They may be feeling like their life is out of their control – if you give them knowledge you give them a way to have control over the most important part of their lives – the food they eat.   And remember, we are all human. Mistakes will happen. Be prepared and learn what to do to ease the symptoms BEFORE it happens. If you make a mistake, it's ok. It may help you to be more careful the next time.

I was first introduced to the gluten-free lifestyle over three years ago with my youngest granddaughter. I was diagnosed with Celiac disease almost two years ago. Three more of my grandchildren (all in the same family) were diagnosed with Celiac disease a few months ago. I have read thousands of ingredient lists; spent countless hours researching on the internet; read hundreds of books about Celiac disease and gluten and wheat. My life revolves around gluten-free. Not a day goes by that I don't think about gluten in some way. You would think I have enough experience with the Celiac lifestyle, gluten-free foods and ingredient lists that I wouldn't make any mistakes, right? Wrong. I live in a combination household – one gluten eater, one gluten-free eater. I manage to get cross-contaminated about once every two months. I suffer the symptoms of nausea, diarrhea, gas pains, swollen joints, migraines and brain fog. When the fog lifts I remind myself to be more careful and to pay more attention to where my food is placed, next time. And about two months later I go through it all over again. It happens.

You need to realize that since gluten is invisible to the naked eye, you won't be able to tell if it's on your counter (the gluten-eater puts their wheat bread on the counter and forgets to wash it), in your shampoo (I accidentally used a shampoo with hydrolyzed wheat protein and got the shampoo in my eye which resulted in an eye infection the required antibiotic eye drops to heal), or on the cookie sheet (I forgot to use parchment paper on the cookie sheet we share). You will probably be contaminated by gluten at some point. Unless you choose to live in a bubble, completely separated from the rest of the world, there will be gluten around you. Accept it, deal with it if you get contaminated and move on. Don't live in fear of gluten. It's there. It's going to get us once in a while. And life goes on.

Denial

The thought of having to change the way you live and the foods you eat may immediately take you down the road to denial. Or you may experience denial after a few months of eating gluten-free. You're feeling better, your symptoms have gone away. You may tell yourself it must be something else. Maybe you have a virus and it will go away if you wait long enough. Your child looks and acts healthier, so maybe he doesn't really have Celiac disease. You may be tempted to "test" gluten at this stage. Maybe "just a little" won't hurt. It's possible that you or your child may not have a physical reaction at this stage because your body has started to heal. This may cause you to question if you really have Celiac disease or if you can eat gluten, again. If you have been eating gluten-free for a few weeks to a few months, the villi has had time to start healing. It can take up to 6 weeks for the villi to recover – each time you eat gluten. Don't let this take you farther down the road to denial. If you start eating gluten again, or sneaking a little here or there, you will eventually become sick again and will need to start the process all over again. It really isn't worth it. You need to continue to eat gluten-free to stay healthy and stop the damage gluten can cause to your intestinal tract.

Anger

Once you've recovered from the denial of your situation and accept that you do, indeed, have Celiac disease, you may experience anger. Anger at doctors who didn't know what was wrong with you or your child and "made" you go through years of pain and numerous symptoms. Remember that doctors are only human. There is no way for them to automatically know what is wrong with us. The symptoms of Celiac disease are similar to the symptoms of so many other health conditions, including the flu.

I experienced symptoms such as severe diarrhea, abdominal cramps, nausea, migraines, rashes and painful swollen joints off and on for 30 years before I started questioning my symptoms. I thought some of these symptoms were caused by illnesses, lactose intolerance or were just a part of getting older. I had injured my knees many times over the years, so I assumed the arthritis was caused by this and the fact that I was getting older. I had lived with migraines since I was in my 20's, so they were just a normal part of my life. I used to think I would break out in a rash (inside the forearm, across the chest or abdomen, or on my face – whenever I was nervous. Of course, I couldn't' explain them when I WASN'T nervous so I would tell myself I must be nervous even though I wasn't aware of it. (That doesn't make a lot of sense, but it was the only explanation I could come up with.) One time my rash covered my body from my neck to my knees, and was so painful and sensitive that I couldn't bear to have my clothes touch my skin. When I went to the doctor, they couldn't tell me what caused it, but gave me some cortisone cream to put on it. (The cream made it worse, by the way. I wonder if it contained gluten?)

A few months before I was diagnosed, I thought I was having a bad winter and was getting the flu over and over again. I didn't realize how serious it was until a co-worker asked me if anything was wrong with me because I had lost so much weight in such a short time. I would "get the flu" for a couple of days and then recover. It would be back within a week and I would go through the diarrhea, vomiting and fever all over again. This was during a very stressful period in my life, so I thought maybe the symptoms were just from all the stress.

Some people may feel anger at God or Fate for allowing this to happen, not knowing what you or your child did to deserve this terrible fate. You need to remember you didn't get Celiac disease because of anything you did. You don't get Celiac disease because you are being punished for something. You get Celiac disease because someone in your ancestral tree had the genetic marker for Celiac disease and passed it on to you.

Children may get angry at their parents and caregivers because their favorite foods have been taken away from them. They may feel like you're punishing them. You make them eat unfamiliar foods with strange names and sometimes strange (to their taste buds) flavors. When they eat an old familiar food (whether accidentally or intentionally) they get sick again and have to suffer through their symptoms. If it's confusing for adults, think how confusing and scary it can be for a child.

Many people get angry at food and personal care manufacturers for seemingly putting gluten in just about everything. Or for using so many names for wheat, rye and barley that you feel like you need to be a scientist to read an ingredient list. Some people even get angry at their friends and family because they can still eat gluten. Or they get angry at their family and friends because they just don't seem to understand how difficult living gluten-free can be.

I've been told (by gluten-eaters) that switching to gluten-free should be easy because "it's just food." What they don't seem to understand that "just food" is a large part of our lives. In addition to nutrition, food can give us comfort and enjoyment and, unfortunately, pain. Food brings families together with evening meals, picnics, family gatherings and holidays. Food brings friends together in restaurants and get-togethers. Business meetings and seminars involve foods. A large part of our lives revolves around food.

I lived with a Celiac grandchild for two years before being diagnosed, myself. I thought I understood the gluten-free lifestyle. I had researched the disease and gluten, itself. I knew how to read an ingredient list. I knew how to avoid cross-contamination. Yet, I made plenty of mistakes for myself during the first few months of changing to a gluten-free lifestyle. Unless you live a gluten-free lifestyle on a daily basis, it's difficult to understand the complexity of it.

Instead of getting angry with people, try to teach them. Explain what Celiac disease is and how it can damage our bodies if we continue to eat foods that contain gluten. If you understand that anger is a normal part of the process of accepting that we DO have Celiac disease may help you get through this stage.

Grief

You or your child may experience grief over all the foods you can no longer eat. You may feel sad because you feel your child will be "different" or will be singled out. You will probably experience the "I can't have ***** anymore" (insert favorite gluten food) many times. You can feel sad for the loss of certain foods, but you need to remember you can still have chicken nuggets and spaghetti and cookies and bread and cake. The specific food can still be eaten – you just need to prepare them a little differently with a few different ingredients. No, you can't have McDonald's Chicken Nuggets. But you CAN learn to make your own. You can either learn to make your own favorite foods, or buy those already prepared – as long as you buy the foods that are gluten-free. With so many manufacturers adding gluten-free items these days, there are many more choices available today than there were just five or ten years ago.

Self-Pity

There are times you may feel sorry for yourself or your child. Poor me, or my poor child – we can't lead a "normal" life anymore. We're different. We aren't like "other people." No one else I know has to do this. I can't just drive through a fast food restaurant to grab something for lunch. It takes longer to prepare a meal than opening a box of packaged food. I have to read ingredient lists before I, or my child, can eat anything.

It's ok to feel sad because you can't have your favorite foods any longer. They are gone and you will miss them. You can feel sorry for yourself, just don't get so caught up in the self-pity that you spend more time feeling sorry for yourself than you do living your life. In our house, we allow self-pity parties – for 10 minutes. We can whine and complain and cry if we need to. We can remember all the foods we can't have and allow ourselves to feel deprived. For 10 minutes. When the short self-pity party is over, we get back to living our life. Allowing ourselves to feel bad is a sort of release. It's difficult to be strong all the time and keep your chin up and just accept this drastic change in our lives without complaint. So, go ahead. Have your pity party. Feel bad, whine, cry if you feel the need. But keep the "party" to a minimum – 10 minutes seems to work for us. It isn't long enough for others to get tired of hearing us whine. If we cry, no one has to worry about how to make us stop – they know it will be over in 10 minutes. If you let the "party" go on any longer, it gets habit forming and can take over your life. Why spend so much time feeling bad, when there are so many positives in life?

We had a positive wall when my granddaughter was first diagnosed. Each day we wrote down one thing that we were thankful for, that made us smile, that produced a positive emotion. Things like, "I told my friend a joke and made her laugh" and "I'm glad I have my eyesight and hearing" and "I love my family" and "The rain was nice today." The positive wall was in the living room where everyone had to look at the positive comments every day. It helped us to stay focused and not to fall into an endless self-pity party. I keep a positive wall at work, now. If I'm feeling the effects of gluten contamination or if I'm wishing I could go through a drive-through and get a hamburger on a soft, white, wheat bun – I read my wall. And I remember how blessed I am and how grateful I am for all the wonderful things I DO have in my life.

Instead of feeling sorry, be thankful. Be thankful you need to read ingredient lists. You know what you're eating now. You may have been unaware of all the additives and chemicals you were eating before switching to gluten-free. You're probably eating more fresh fruits and vegetables which is certainly healthier. You're taking the time to prepare your own meals from scratch which is better for you than eating additive and chemical-laden pre-packaged foods. Perhaps a family member has been tested for Celiac disease because of yours or your child's diagnosis and discovered they too need to eat gluten-free and are on their way to becoming healthier. Be thankful for that.

Guilt

If you or your child accidently eats a food that contains gluten, or eats a food that has been cross-contaminated, you may feel guilty for causing the reactions that follow. We are all human and there is always room for human error. No one is perfect and accidents will happen. I have been gluten-free for almost two years myself, and have dealt with the gluten-free lifestyle for almost 4 years because of my youngest grandchild. And I still make mistakes. When it happens to me, I think back to what I have eaten, what surface my food touched, where the food was manufactured – to try to figure out what made me sick. I suffer the consequences and move forward. Life goes on. You try to do better in the future, but accept that mistakes can be made. Considering 1 in 133 people have Celiac disease, you know you're not alone.

Acceptance

Acceptance is the final stage. You will learn to accept your diagnosis and that this change in what you eat will continue for the rest of your life. Turning a product over and reading the ingredient list before buying anything will become second nature to you. Preparing many of your own foods, instead of driving through a fast food restaurant or preparing pre-packaged foods will become "normal". Once you begin to feel better and do not have to deal with the old symptoms, you will realize the gluten-free lifestyle is a better choice.

Don't worry if you experience this myriad of emotions more than once. This is normal, too. I find myself walking past a bakery and smell the fresh baked bread and see the rolls and donuts and cookies – and say to myself, "Oh, I wish I could eat those." And then I remember what will happen to me if I do, and the desire to eat all those wheat products promptly disappears.

Support Groups

Having a good support system, whether family, friends or other Celiacs, is very important. It helps to have others who understand your new gluten-free lifestyle. There are many Celiac support groups available across the country. Support groups are great for meeting other people who live the same lifestyle that you do. They understand the frustrations and symptoms and the day to day challenges. Support groups are also a great resource for new recipes, information on the latest Celiac research and just meeting new friends. If you can't find a support group near you, start one. You may be surprised at the number of people who need to eat gluten-free that live in your area.

Attitude and Choices

The key to living with your gluten-free lifestyle is in your attitude. Life is a series of choices. Each choice we make has a consequence. How we deal with these consequences determines the direction our life will take. Our choices control how we feel; if we are happy or sad; if we are feeling sorry for ourselves; if we are blaming someone or something else for where our life is at; if we are rejoicing in a new day, a new sunrise, the laughter of a child, the smile of a friend. Instead of looking at a situation as something bad that is happening to us, look at it as a new opportunity. An opportunity to learn about new ingredients; an opportunity to teach someone about Celiac disease; an opportunity to choose to be healthier. Every situation can be viewed as negative or positive. Go for the positive.

The phrase "It can always be worse" really is true. No matter how bad you think your situation is, it could really be worse. There are always others who are dealing with things that are worse than what we are living with at any moment. Be thankful and grateful for what you have. Celiac disease can be challenging, frustrating and cause us to be sick at times. But Celiac disease doesn't make us lose our limbs or eyesight or hearing, we don't have to take bottles of medications on a daily basis, we don't need chemotherapy to treat it. All we need to do is change the foods we eat and we can become healthy. Put into perspective, that doesn't seem so bad, does it?

Each day, we are given a new sunrise; the warmth of the sun; the bite of the cold; another day with our family and friends. Life shouldn't be about "I can't . . ." Life IS about "**I am!** – I am alive."

WILL I EVER BE "Normal"?

? ? ?

Will I Ever Be "Normal"?

A fellow Celiac mentioned the other day that they would just like to lead a "normal" life. I started thinking about what is "normal"? When we say we want to lead a "normal" life, or we want to be a "normal" person, or we want "normal" kids — what exactly do we mean? Do we mean we want to be "like everyone else"? Is everyone except me "normal"? Does that mean that everyone except me is exactly the same which translates into normal? Am I the only person who isn't "normal"? Or do we mean we want to live without issues? Do we want to live without dietary issues, without behavioral issues, without financial issues, without stress issues, etc.? If you stop to think about how our lives would actually be without any "issues", that translates into BORING. DULL. ENDLESS.

Without the lows of "issues" we wouldn't be able to experience any highs. Without negatives, we wouldn't know what a positive feels like. There would be nothing to compare anything to. How do we appreciate the good things in our lives if we have no bad things to compare them to? How do we experience happy if we have no sad at the opposite end? How could we anticipate a new day and all the wonderful things it might bring, if each day was "normal" and the same as yesterday and the day before and tomorrow and next week and on and on and on.

Switching to a gluten-free lifestyle has certainly had its issues. But it's also been a wonderful learning experience. I've learned things I never considered before going gluten-free and have discovered you're really never too old to learn something new each day. I learned you can live without wheat, rye and barley. When they make you sick, a "whole grain" diet really isn't better for you. You don't need wheat bread to make sandwiches, French toast or bread pudding. I discovered the term "flour" is a generalization. I learned you can use flours made from rice, tapioca, almonds, potatoes and quinoa. (Before going gluten-free, I had never even heard of quinoa and certainly couldn't pronounce it! Now I can bake with it.)

I have expanded my vocabulary by learning new words like Spelt, Triticale, Semolina, Maltose and Hydroxypropyltrimonium (I can even pronounce that one now.) My ability to "Google" has increased ten-fold. I've learned to take the information I find with a grain of salt – and to realize that some of the information doesn't hold true for each and every person, no matter how "normal" we think we are. What is good for the goose is not always good for the gander, so to speak.

The way I shop for groceries has been a definite learning experience. I discovered sections of the grocery store I never knew existed. There are all sorts of new foods waiting for me to discover them, quietly calling my name from the bottom shelf in some semi-lit aisle. Now that I take more time shopping, I've come to enjoy my local grocery stores and natural foods stores. I used to buy most of my groceries at the same store, week after week. I have expanded my horizons and have ventured out to new stores and new cities looking for more gluten-free options. I consider the grocery store my second home. Different stores have different gluten-free options and very different prices. I used to be able to shop for a week's worth of groceries in under 20 minutes. Now, I may take an hour or more. I take my time, I read every ingredient list on every item I consider purchasing. By slowing down, I've had the chance to have conversations with fellow shoppers, discovered new foods and invented new recipes standing in an aisle in the grocery store. I know I'm eating healthier be4cause I buy more fresh fruits and vegetables and I buy fewer chemical-laden packaged foods.

I would like to say my handwriting has improved from all the product names and manufacturing companies I've written down for future research, but I believe what has improved is my ability to read my own handwriting. I read a lot more of it, lately. If I'm unsure of the ingredient in a particular product, I will write down the name of the product, the size, the ingredient in question and the company that manufactures it. Once I am home again, I will research all of the above on the internet. If I still can't find the answers I'm looking for, I will call the company directly.

I'm saving more money now. The amount of money I spend on eating out has been greatly reduced. I rarely eat in restaurants these days. Many restaurants have jumped on the gluten-free bandwagon in an effort to increase sales and attract more customers. They advertise they now offer gluten-free options – foods with no gluten IN THE INGREDIENTS. Unfortunately, many of them don't understand the danger of cross-contamination or the consequence of eating a gluten-free item that was placed on the same preparation table as something that contains wheat. They don't understand if their cook picks up a wheat hamburger bun and then puts lettuce in a salad bowl for their gluten-free customer, that customer is going to become very sick.

Learning to cook – or perhaps I should say RE-learning to cook – has given me a new understanding of various ingredients. I now know what certain ingredients do, why you use them, and what happens if you forget to add them to your recipe. (I learned this the hard way.) I am able to convert recipes that I made for years, that contained gluten ingredients, into gluten-free recipes and they taste good! Which means my math skills have improved – converting, measuring, adding, multiplying – what a great positive.

Eating foods that are good for me allows me to enjoy my day to day life more. When I don't have to deal with diarrhea, migraines, nausea or joints so swollen I can't walk, on a daily basis, I can enjoy the changing hues of the sunrise or the laughter of a child. I can take the time to watch a hawk glide and soar above me, searching for his next meal (which I'm sure will also be gluten-free.)

My group of friends and "family" has increased in the past two years. I have met so many wonderful people since changing to a gluten-free lifestyle. People in grocery stores, fellow Celiacs on Facebook and manufacturers and distributors of gluten-free products. These people are friendly, open and willing to offer information and support. I would never have met these new "family" members had I not changed to a gluten-free lifestyle.

Life is good and much better now that I'm gluten-free. Life is NOT the same as it was and I see that as a good thing. Life is about choices – and consequences. Every choice we make in our lives comes with a consequence. How we deal with the consequences determines which direction our life will take. We all live with the consequences of our choices. Changing to a gluten-free lifestyle has had many wonderful consequences. So, is my life "normal"? Yes – normal FOR ME.

INFANTS AND CELIAC DISEASE

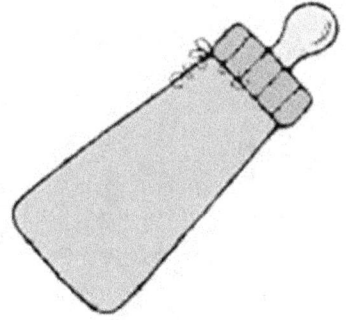

Infants and Celiac Disease

It is difficult to diagnose Celiac disease in infants because of their size and inability to tell us when something is wrong. Symptoms may develop within 2 – 3 months after solid foods are introduced into their diet. Babies normally double their birth weight in the first six months. They should triple their birth weight within the first year.

Slow weight gain and stunted growth can be an indication of Celiac disease. My daughter has seven children, four of whom have been diagnosed with Celiac disease. The three children with the most severe reaction to gluten were slow to increase weight as babies. All of them had problems with diarrhea, diaper rash and vomiting after eating as babies. The youngest had diaper rash so severe it would bleed. The saying, "hindsight is 20/20" is true. We can look back to issues they had as babies and now say "I bet gluten was the cause of this symptom."

Symptoms, in addition to slow weight gain, that may indicate Celiac disease in infants can include the following:

> Severe diarrhea
> Projectile vomiting
> Anemia
> Irritable, cranky, colicky
> Lethargic
> Whining/crying for no apparent reason
> Hives
> Severe diaper rash
> Abdominal cramps
> > (pulling legs up combined with painful cry)
> High fever
> Dehydration

Symptoms may appear before they begin eating solid foods. Many infant formulas contain wheat and/or gluten. Studies have shown high levels of gliadin in breast milk. (Gliadin is the protein in gluten that causes the immune system to react.) Whatever the mother eats DOES pass through the breast milk to her child.

When infants experience intestinal problems or are colicky, their pediatrician my recommend the mother remove certain foods from her diet. Foods which can be passed through her breast milk to her child. Typical foods that are removed are dairy, beans and eggs. Very rarely will a doctor recommend the mother remove wheat and foods that contain gluten. Many children who were fussy, colicky babies are later diagnosed with Celiac disease.

CHILDREN AND CELIAC DISEASE

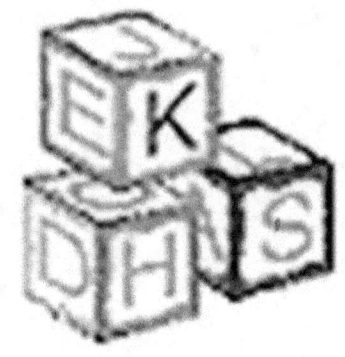

Children and Celiac Disease

School age children who receive a diagnosis of Celiac disease or gluten sensitivity have their own set of difficulties that are different from the difficulties that babies, small children, teens and older adults go through. Until they reach school, they are basically in a controlled situation. They are either with their parents or with someone who takes care of them while the parents work. They are also young enough to believe the adults are smart and know everything. They start to outgrow this belief once they start school and get that first taste of independence and freedom.

School starts their journey to independence. They will be making decisions for themselves in a place where there is no mom or dad to tell them what they should do. At school, they can share their lunch with their friends, they have snacks provided by the school or other parents and there is usually food for birthdays and holiday celebrations. These are all places where your child is allowed to choose what they will eat. They are also places where it is easy to cross-contaminate gluten-free foods.

Once a child reaches school age, they make more friends. Friends who want them to come to their house to play, or to sleep over, or for a birthday party. This means that not only do you and your child need to understand Celiac disease and the foods that are safe, but so do your child's friends and the parents of your child's friends.

Education is the key to living a gluten-free lifestyle, no matter what your age is. It is very important that the child with Celiac disease understand what it is, what it can do to their body if they continue to eat gluten, and how make informed choices in the foods they eat. Teach them to be self-sufficient and independent. If they are dependent on the adults around them to be able to tell them what they should eat, they're going to be sick a lot of the time. Many people don't know what Celiac disease is. And the same number people don't know what gluten is. If they don't know what gluten is, they can't tell your child if the food he is about to eat contains it.

When you child will be visiting a friend's house, you need to talk to the other child's parents ahead of time. Explain what Celiac disease is, the need to avoid gluten and what possible reactions your child may experience if they do eat foods with gluten. Rather than giving the other parents a long list of foods your child CAN'T have, offer to send "safe" food along with your child. Your child should know ahead of time what foods are safe for them to eat, so they can make informed choices for themselves.

Birthday parties can be a challenge for children who need to avoid gluten. A regular birthday cake is off-limits for your child. You can send gluten-free cupcakes with your child so they can still enjoy having cake with the other children. Talk to the parent ahead of time about other snacks that may be served at birthday party. Give them a list of foods that are safe for your child, or offer to bring additional snacks to the party, that will be safe for your child.

TEENAGERS AND CELIAC DISEASE

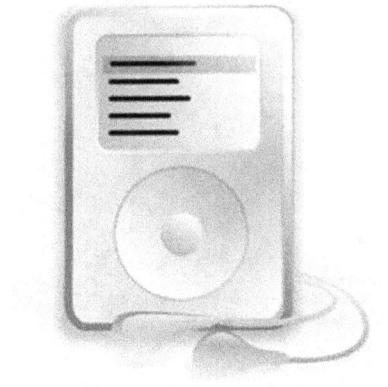

Teenagers and Celiac Disease

Regardless of a person's age when they are diagnosed with Celiac disease or gluten sensitivity, we all have one thing in common – gluten destroys our small intestine and can lead to other health issues.

Teenagers with Celiac disease face their own set of issues that is different from small children or adults. Adolescence is a time of growing. They are growing physically, mentally and emotionally. Peer pressure is probably the strongest influence during adolescence than at any other time in our lives. Teenagers want to "fit in" with their friends, be considered part of a group and few want to stand out as being "different". Teenagers who tend to be on the shy side, may be afraid their Celiac disease may draw attention to them and put them in the spotlight.

Anyone who has raised a teenager knows about mood changes! Hormones are running rampant and can change a sweet, good-natured child into a grunting, sloppy, bored creature from some unknown planet. This isn't just teenagers with Celiac disease – this is ALL teenagers.

When you add Celiac disease to all of these raging hormones, it can become a difficult situation for a teenager. Educating your teenager and teaching them to accept Celiac disease as just another of life's challenges may help.

Due to the body's inability to absorb nutrients, because of damaged villi in the small intestine, teenagers may experience levels of low energy or fatigue. They may feel as though they just don't have enough energy to do simple things. It takes a lot of energy for your body to battle gluten. My 13-year old granddaughter has told me when she has accidentally eaten something with gluten in it or has been cross-contaminated, she feels like all she's wrung out, like a wet dish rag. It's hard to find the energy to get up and do anything. When she sits in a chair (whether it's at home or at school), she falls asleep. It's as though your body is taking control and is telling you, "Hey, I need time to regenerate. I'm shutting down and going to sleep and I don't care where you are." It seems to take all of her energy to fight the gluten and there isn't any energy left for walking or talking or staying awake.

Everyone gets frustrated at one time or another. With gluten contamination, however, you seem to be frustrated by the smallest, insignificant things. Your reaction is not proportionate to the situation that is causing your frustration. Under normal circumstances, if you have difficulty opening a jar of peanut butter, you may ask for help or tap the jar on the counter to loosen it. When you've been contaminated by gluten, it's an entirely different story. When the cover won't turn, you get frustrated, you yell, you may feel like crying and are tempted to throw the jar across the room. It's hard to control your emotions at this time.

Hormones can cause teenagers to have mood swings, but hormones may not be the cause of all of your teenager's mood swings. Gluten can also be the cause of mood swings, depression and behavioral problems such as hyperactivity and anger issues. When my 10-year old grandson is contaminated by gluten he experiences drastic mood swings. He's happy one minute and becomes a frustrated, angry child five minutes later. Simple everyday situations such as cleaning his room or scraping his dinner plate can bring on tears, frustration and angry outbursts.

Celiac teens may complain about constant hunger and appear to eat one meal per day – starting the moment they get up in the morning and continuing until they go to bed at night. There seems to be a bottomless pit inside that never gets full. When the villi in the small intestine are damaged and flattened, they aren't able to absorb the nutrients needed for a growing teenager. This causes the "I'm starving" feeling. They eat plenty of healthy food, but the nutrients are not being absorbed along the way.

Gluten can also cause headaches and migraines, neither of which are pleasant to deal with. The headaches don't seem to respond well to pain medication. They seem to last until the gluten is out of your body. Migraines are much more painful. Bright lights and everyday noises can cause excruciating pain. I have found that drinking plenty of water to help flush the gluten from your system helps somewhat. Before my youngest granddaughter was diagnosed with Celiac disease, she experienced headaches from gluten. Since she was only 14 months old, she couldn't tell us what was wrong. She would cry and scream and pound her fists on the sides of her head, over and over again. This reaction could last from hours to a days.

Teenagers may have problems in school due to intestinal issues, mood swings and brain fog. Bodily functions (such as vomiting, gas and diarrhea) are not subjects most teens care to discuss with others. The need to use the bathroom frequently can be embarrassing, especially if they need to leave during class. Many times, it's just not possible to wait until class is over, or until lunch time. Regular attendance may be affected by gluten. An intestinal reaction, combined with fatigue and/or headaches, may cause teenagers to miss more school than normal. Most schools allow a certain number of "sick" days, which teenagers with Celiac disease could exceed. It's a good idea to talk with your child's teachers and the school nurse to explain the reactions your child may experience if they consume gluten. Explain to them why your child may miss more school than other teens.

The inability to concentrate, fatigue and brain fog can play havoc with a teen's grades. Comprehension may be difficult. It can be frustrating when they understood a math problem one day and two days later can't remember how to perform the same calculation. It's even more frustrating when you can't remember what you were taught 15 minutes later. Fatigue can wear a person down very quickly. It seems like everything takes so much effort to accomplish. It's embarrassing when you can't keep your eyes open during class and you seem to fall asleep every time you sit still for five minutes. The inattentiveness and brain fog my cause some teachers to assume the teen doesn't care or isn't trying hard enough to learn. This can cause even more frustration on the teen's part because they know they're trying – they just can't make their brain function the way they want it to, sometimes.

Other areas that can cause issues for teenagers are class projects, field trips, chemistry & biology class and Home Ec. You need to be sure the items, such as paste, glue and paints used during class projects are gluten-free. The same holds true for projects and experiments in chemistry and biology class. Talk to their teachers and explain why the items need to be gluten-free. Explain the consequences your teen will experience if they are not gluten-free. If they will be using items that contain gluten, discuss alternative options.

Home Ec class, better known today as FACS Class, can pose problems when the students are learning to cook. Airborne particles of wheat flour can cause problems for teens with Celiac disease or a gluten sensitivity. The airborne particles can be inhaled or may cause skin problems such as hives, blisters and DH (Dermatitis Herpetiformis). Your teen should not be removed from the class, but there may be alternative ingredients that can be used. Perhaps having your teen wear rubber gloves during the food preparation would be a solution. It would be educational for the class to learn to prepare gluten-free foods on occasion.

There are many situations where cross-contamination can occur. Sharing food and water/pop bottles is obvious, but may happen. Learning to live a gluten-free lifestyle is an ongoing learning experience. Many times we do things because of habit. We're used to doing and eating certain things, that we automatically do them over and over again. Shortly after my 13-year old granddaughter, Morgan, was diagnosed, she was contaminated by a shared water bottle. She brought her own gluten-free lunch to school and was careful not to contaminate it with anyone else's food. But, when her friend asked if she could have a drink from Morgan's water bottle, she automatically agreed. Unfortunately, the friend had been eating a sandwich made with wheat bread. There was enough gluten left on the mouth of the bottle to contaminate my granddaughter and make her sick for two days.

Another area that teens (and adults) may not consider is dating. Kissing, in particular. Depending on what the other person has eaten or had to drink, prior to sharing a kiss, could create a situation for contamination. A cookie or a cracker will leave gluten on a person's lips, teeth and tongue. This doesn't mean they shouldn't kiss at all, it just means both partners need to be careful. Brushing teeth is an excellent way to remove gluten from the mouth and teeth.

Interview with Morgan (teenage Celiac)

Morgan is a teenager who has Celiac disease. She was diagnosed 3 months ago, but has been living with a little sister who has Celiac disease for the past 3 ½ years. Like many of us who live with someone who has Celiac disease, she thought she knew enough about the disease and the gluten-free food and how to avoid cross-contamination. And like many of us who are diagnosed later, she discovered gluten-free is a whole new world when you have to live it for yourself instead of just live it WITH someone.

Morgan has a very positive attitude about her diagnosis. It's here, it won't go away, so accept it and learn to live with it. Don't fight it. There is more to life than the food you eat.

I asked Morgan a few questions to help her tell us her point of view on being diagnosed with Celiac disease:

1. How did you feel when you first found out you have Celiac disease?

I felt like I was going to be made fun of for being different, and I knew I couldn't have all my favorite foods, anymore, so I had to think of new foods. I have to learn to convert everything to GF. I had to watch out for not only food, but lotions, tooth paste, mouth wash, shampoo, etc.

2. Was it hard to change to GF foods?

At first it was hard but now it's getting easier day by day. You have to keep the saying "take it one day at a time, it WILL get easier" in your head.

3. What symptoms went away after changing to gluten-free foods?

I didn't feel like throwing up all the time, I didn't have constant headaches, my belly didn't hurt daily, and I wasn't bloated all the time.

4. What difficulties do you have at home now that you're GF?

I have to worry about not cross contaminating myself.

5. What difficulties do you have at school now that you're GF?

When I'm eating lunch I can't set my food down or I will get sick. I have to worry about the soap in the bathrooms.

6. Are there classes at school (not lunch) that you find it hard to be GF?

Yes. FACS – where we cook food with gluten in it.

7. What things do you do at school to stay safe from gluten?

I do not set my food down at lunch.

8. Do your friends understand Celiac disease?

Some of them do. Some don't care. Some just don't understand it.

9. Do your friends understand cross-contamination?

One or two of them. The others don't think of it.

10. How do you explain Celiac disease to others?

I can't have anything with wheat, rye, or barley in it. If you put something that has any of that in it on the counter and I put my food there, I can no longer eat it.

11. What do you do to stay safe when you stay at a friend's house?

Bring my own food.

12. What do you do if your friends want you to eat at a restaurant or fast food place?

I don't eat, and just watch them.

13. What school functions do you find difficult?

Umm..That's a tough one. football games and school dances for sure, because they have food I can't have so I have to wait until I get home to eat anything.

14. Do you feel different than other teenagers? How do you handle that?

Yes, I feel different. I just go with it. If you don't like it, don't look.

15. Are you tempted to cheat and eat gluten foods?

Yes, all the time, but then I remember the pain factor and what happens when I eat it.

16. What do you do to keep from cheating?

Think about the consequences.

17. What is the hardest part of living gluten-free?

Not being able to do what everyone else does. Not being able to eat out anymore. Not being able to just grab a candy bar at the checkout. etc.

18. What advice do you have for other teenagers who have just been diagnosed and are having difficulties?

Don't cheat. It will NOT be worth it. And don't care what other people think of you. It's good to be different.

ADULTS AND CELIAC DISEASE

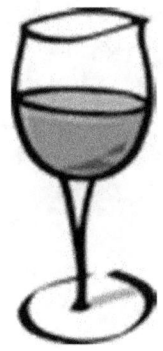

Adults and Celiac Disease

People who are diagnosed with Celiac disease or a gluten sensitivity as an adult have their own set of issues. I, myself, was diagnosed at 56. I had many, many years of symptoms that were either misdiagnosed or were considered just part of "getting older".

I also had many, many years of eating foods that contained gluten, never realizing that the food I was eating was what was making me sick. We all develop favorite foods and comfort foods throughout our lives. My main comfort food was homemade bread. Homemade wheat bread. My mother made bread while I was growing up. The warm, yeasty smell of fresh bread filled our kitchen on a weekly basis. As soon as the first loaf would come out of the oven, nice and warm and crusty and smelling wonderful, my mother would cut off both ends of the loaf and slather them with butter. Fresh, warm bread is something I associated with happy times with my mother.

I continued this "sharing the bread" with my children. On those cold Minnesota winter days, I would bake a loaf or two of fresh bread. The kitchen would fill with the yeasty smell of comfort. My daughters and I would share the crusty ends of the loaf as soon as we pulled them from the oven.

When I first began my gluten-free lifestyle, I discovered that packaged gluten-free bread didn't quite compare with packaged wheat bread. Homemade gluten-free bread wasn't quite the same as homemade wheat bread. Learning to bake with gluten-free ingredients takes time and experience. Thankfully, I'm not easily discourage and am willing to keep trying until I feel I'm successful. Many a loaf of gluten-free bread (better known as bricks) were tossed out before I developed a recipe and a process that worked well each time. I can again enjoy my warm, crusty comfort food moments with fresh bread right out of the oven.

I was diagnosed at an age where I knew what wheat products tasted like. I had my favorites. There were meals that I cooked more often than others such as pizza, lasagna, hamburgers on wheat buns, tacos, turkey with stuffing, cookies, cakes and pastries. They all used wheat flour. I can still have all of those foods, I just need to use gluten-free ingredients and prepare them a little differently. Almost two years later, I have them pretty much down pat. But it was definitely a learning experience. I learned you really aren't too old to learn something new!

This is not to say it was an easy transition. I experienced the loss of certain foods (and still experience this loss from time to time.) I experienced the "why me" syndrome. I experienced the anger at needing to drastically change my life at this late stage in the game. I learned that I had been an impulse shopper. Grabbing freshly baked rolls, or cookies or breads from the bakery aisle just because they looked good and I was in the mood for something sweet, or yeasty was the norm for me. Picking up a bag of chips or a candy bar or two at the checkout just because it was there and the line was slow occurred more often than I would like to admit. I have discovered my impulse shopping has dropped dramatically – mainly because there are fewer gluten-free items available compared to items that contain gluten. Certain products are put in specific places in stores to encourage us to impulse shop. Those products no longer call my name, because the consequences I will experience if eat them outweigh the temporary pleasure I might receive from eating them. Foods on the end caps of aisles and all those small, inexpensive items that surround the checkouts just don't interest me anymore.

Eating out has been the biggest hurdle since going gluten-free. Not that I ate out a lot when I was eating foods that contained gluten. But the option was always there. If I wanted to, I could stop and pick up a pizza on my way home. If I wanted to, I could go through the drive-thru of the local fast food restaurant. If I wanted to, I could go out to lunch with my co-workers, or meet friends for dinner after work. All I had to worry about what which item on the menu I wanted to eat.

I can still do all of those things, if I want to. However, there is a little more planning involved with each situation. I can still stop and pick up a pizza on my way home – as long as I stop at the pizza place that offers gluten-free pizzas that are individually wrapped off-site and I make sure they bake my pizza on a pan, not directly in the oven where all the pizzas with wheat flour are baked. I also need to be sure the kitchen staff puts on new gloves before unwrapping and handling my gluten-free pizza. Personally, I find it's easier to buy the gluten-free ingredients and make my own pizza at home.

I can still go through the local fast food restaurant on my way home. I choose to go inside now, where I can watch how they prepare my food and make sure they put on clean gloves before handling my food. I know which items are safe and which are not (mainly through trial and error.) Just because one location of a particular fast food restaurant has foods that are safe and they know how to prepare my gluten-free food doesn't mean I trust a different location of the same fast food chain. Gluten-free safety is dependent upon the people who are preparing it and how much training and education on safe gluten-free foods they have received.

I can still go out to lunch and dinner with friends. However, I now need to find out what restaurant we are going to ahead of time. I need to know if they offer gluten-free options, how they prepare the gluten-free foods and how informed the kitchen staff and servers are about cross-contamination. If the chosen restaurant doesn't offer gluten-free foods, I need to know which of their meals could be prepared to be gluten-free. (I eat a lot of salads at restaurants.) I also need to discuss the selection of the restaurant with the friends I plan to meet. It's time-consuming and, at times, frustrating. But it is also necessary if I want to stay healthy. It has certainly cut down on the amount of money I spend on eating out.

Living a gluten-free lifestyle takes time and effort. "Gluten-free" is something we need to be aware of on a daily basis. There is no time when you can just forget that you need to stay gluten-free.

Considering the consequences we will experience if we are not diligent, it's well worth the extra time and effort.

Food is not the only area where we need to be concerned with gluten-free products. Personal care items such as soap, shampoo, conditioner, hair products, lotions and make-up also need to be gluten-free. Knowledge is the key. Research your favorite products to find out if they're gluten-free. Many products are gluten-free but do not state "gluten-free" on the labels. Read the ingredients, check out the manufacturer's websites or call the company directly to ask if their products contain gluten or are manufactured on the same lines as products that contain gluten. If your favorite products are not safe, research other products that state they are gluten-free. Google is a great resource. If you type in "Is *** (insert brand name product) gluten-free?" you will find many websites that will offer information. Remember to check more than one source for verification. Unfortunately, there is also a lot of conflicting information on the internet. Check reliable sources such as www.celiac.com, and read comments and opinions from numerous users.

If you work outside the home, it is a good idea to keep non-perishable gluten-free foods at your desk. Business meetings can sometimes include rolls, donuts or other foods that contain gluten. Gluten-free crackers, pretzels and cookies can be kept at your desk for those last-minute meetings and breaks. Business lunches can still be attended if you prepare ahead of time. Find out the name of the restaurant the meeting is to be held at. Call the restaurant and ask if they offer gluten-free choices. If they don't have specific gluten-free options, ask about foods that could be prepared to be gluten-free. Be sure to discuss the dangers of cross-contamination.

Changing you're the foods you eat and the way you live can be challenging as an adult. It's not impossible. Keep in mind if you don't change, you will be putting your health at risk and will continue to cause damage to your body. Not changing your lifestyle can put you at risk for many other serious health issues.

A GLUTEN-FREE KITCHEN

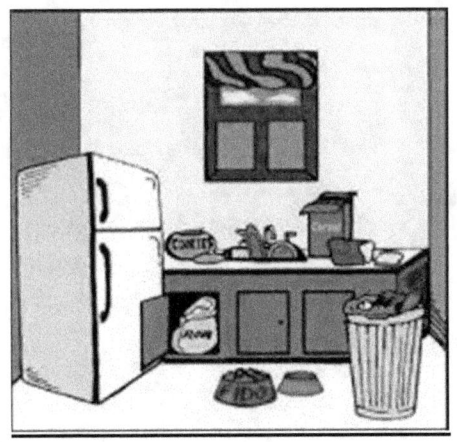

A Gluten-free Kitchen

The easiest way to guarantee that you don't eat gluten, either by eating a food that contains gluten or through cross-contamination from foods that contain gluten, is by making your entire kitchen gluten-free. Remove any and all foods that contain gluten and never let them into your house again. If one or more people in a household need to follow a gluten-free lifestyle, many people choose to have the entire household go gluten-free. Granted, this makes it easier to avoid cross-contamination issues, but it isn't always possible for everyone to make this choice.

Many of us need to keep a "combination kitchen". Some people are gluten-free and some can still eat gluten. If you have a "combination family" – some who eat gluten and some who need to be gluten-free, it is important to have "safe" areas for gluten-free foods. Cross-contamination is easy in a combined kitchen. If you have a combination kitchen, both gluten and gluten-free foods and ingredients, there are a few steps you can take to avoid gluten contamination.

Cupboards

Keeping a separate gluten-free cupboard will help avoid gluten contamination. We have one cupboard that contains only gluten-free foods such as gluten-free flours, gluten-free pasta, gluten-free peanut butter, gluten-free spices, gluten-free cookies and crackers, etc. Nothing that contains gluten is allowed in this cupboard. If you keep your gluten-free flours in their own containers, but store them next to the gluten flours, it is too easy to contaminate them. Unless you wipe off your gluten flour container completely every time you bake (which, I'm sorry, I just don't have time to do when I'm baking) there are enough flour particles on the outside of the container to contaminate your gluten-free flours. If you spill gluten flour on the outside of the container, put it in the cupboard and then pick up your gluten-free container – your hands are contaminated with gluten flour and can contaminate the entire container of gluten-free flour. Because I like to "grab and go" when I bake, I keep my gluten-free ingredients separate. That way I don't have to worry if I touched something with gluten in it before I grab one of my gluten-free ingredients.

Refrigerator

Designate a separate area in the refrigerator for gluten free foods. Any container that requires you to scoop the contents out, such as butter/margarine, mayonnaise, sour cream, cheeses and meats, should be kept separate to be sure it isn't accidentally contaminated. You should also label items such as butter/margarine, mayonnaise, jelly, sour cream, etc. as "gluten-free". We have two containers of mayonnaise – one is labeled gluten-free and the other is not labeled. Our gluten-eaters know they can put their knife (that has touched their wheat bread) in the unlabeled mayonnaise without worrying that the Celiacs will get sick. We also have two containers of margarine and mustard – one is labeled gluten-free. Any container that someone will use a knife or spoon in, we keep separate gluten and gluten-free containers. We have one shelf in the refrigerator that is only for gluten-free foods. The Celiacs know it is safe to eat food on this shelf.

Countertops

Countertops are a good place for cross-contamination. If you set a slice of wheat bread on the counter, remove it and then place a slice of gluten-free bread in the same area, the gluten-free bread is now contaminated with enough gluten to cause a reaction. To keep your counter tops safe, wash them with soapy water before and after preparing gluten-free foods. This doesn't mean just the small center area that most people use, but the entire countertop. Wash all the way to the back and sides and lift up the appliances that sit on the counter. (I specify the entire countertop because I have had to tell children and teenagers that a countertop is the entire surface – not just the middle. It's the same concept I use to explain how to vacuum to my grandchildren.) You never know where a bread crumb may be hiding. Someone may have set a gluten item on the countertop when you weren't there and forgot to wash it with soapy water. We're all human – it's easy to forget, especially when gluten-free and cross-contamination are all new to you. We've been at this for years, and we still make mistakes occasionally.

Pots / Pans / Baking dishes

There is no need to have separate pots, pans or baking dishes for gluten-free foods. A thorough washing in a dishwasher or by hand with plenty of warm, soapy water should remove any gluten from your pans. If you have a small number of pots and pans and need to use the same pan to cook gluten-free foods and foods that contain gluten, you will need to cook the gluten-free foods first, and then the foods that contain gluten. If you use non-stick pans, be sure there is no wearing or chipping of the non-stick surface. If you feel safer using separate pans for gluten and gluten-free foods, by all means purchase another set of pans. However, this can become quite expensive. If you use the same cookie sheets for foods that contain gluten and gluten-free foods, you can keep gluten-free foods safe by covering your cookie sheets with parchment paper when baking gluten-free foods. Remember to wash the cookie sheets thoroughly after each use.

Silverware / Serving utensils

There is no need to have separate silverware and serving utensils for gluten-free foods. A thorough washing in a dishwasher or by hand with plenty of warm, soapy water will remove any gluten from your utensils. Just be sure to keep them separate while serving food. If you put a serving spoon in a gluten food, do not use the same spoon to serve the gluten-free foods.

Plastic containers

If you use plastic containers for storing leftovers, your safest option is to keep separate containers for foods that contain gluten and gluten-free foods. Plastic can absorb gluten and contaminate your gluten-free foods. (Think of tomato sauce – if you store tomato sauce in a plastic container, the container can absorb the tomato and turn orange. I use to have plenty of half white/half orange plastic containers.) Be sure to label the containers for gluten-free foods to avoid using the wrong containers in the future. Use the gluten-free plastic containers ONLY for gluten-free foods. I label mine with a black permanent marker so there is no question as to what was stored in the container last.

Indoor grills (George Foreman)

If you use an indoor grill, such as a George Forman grill, you have two options – (1) Cook all gluten-free foods first, then cook gluten foods and wash thoroughly with warm soapy water when done cooking, or (2) keep two separate grills – one for foods that contain gluten and one for gluten-free foods. Be sure to label each grill to avoid confusion. My George Foreman grill has a non-stick surface, and is easy to clean. Be sure to wash all surfaces and nooks & crannies of the grill after cooking foods that contain gluten. Do not cook gluten-free and gluten foods at the same time on the same grill. Cook the gluten-free foods first.

Toaster

The toaster is one appliance that you should invest in having duplicates. A separate toaster for gluten-free breads is essential. Do not share a toaster with breads that contain gluten. The gluten bread touches the wires inside the toaster and crumbs fall to the bottom, contaminating the toaster. Be sure to label the gluten-free toaster as only gluten-free.

Breadmakers

Do not use the same breadmaker for foods that contain gluten and gluten-free breads. There are many small spaces that can hold gluten if not thoroughly cleaned after baking gluten bread. If you plan to use a breadmaker to make wheat and gluten-free breads, designate one breadmaker to be used only for gluten-free breads and label it clearly.

Cutting boards

Cutting boards – whether plastic or wood – can be another source of cross-contamination. Plastic and wood can absorb gluten and can easily contaminate gluten-free foods. Keep separate cutting boards and either label each one (gluten and gluten-free) or choose a different color for each cutting board.

Colanders (strainers)

It is best to keep separate colanders / strainers for foods that contain gluten and gluten-free foods. If you must share one colander for both types of food, strain the gluten free food first, then the food that contains gluten. Be sure to wash the colander very thoroughly after straining gluten foods, such as pasta. Small pieces of pasta can get stuck in the tiny holes in a colander and contaminate gluten-free foods. We keep separate colanders – purple for gluten-free foods, green for gluten foods.

Oven Racks

If you have ever baked a pizza with a wheat crust directly on your oven rack, your oven rack is contaminated. You have two choices – thoroughly wash the oven racks to be sure there is no trace of gluten on the racks. You will need to do this each time you bake a gluten item directly on the oven rack. Or, you can cover the oven rack with aluminum foil each time you need to bake a gluten-free item directly on the oven rack – such as gluten-free pizza. Personally, I choose the aluminum foil. If I don't have to clean each and every one of the ribs on each of my oven racks, I'm not going to. Aluminum foil is inexpensive and oh so much easier. You can also bake your gluten-free foods on a pan or cookie sheet to protect them from being contaminated by the oven rack.

CELIAC DISEASE AND NUTRITION
~
WHY DEFICIENCIES HAPPEN

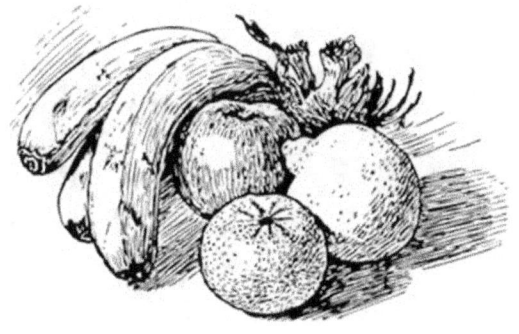

Celiac Disease and Nutrition:
Why Nutritional Deficiencies Happen

When you switch to a gluten-free lifestyle, you stop eating wheat, rye and barley. These grains contain several vitamins and minerals that are essential to a healthy body. Manufacturers are always telling us to eat "whole grain" foods, because these grains help us to stay healthy.

Unfortunately, for Celiacs, some of these grains can be life-threatening. Eating wheat, rye and barley can make us very UNhealthy. Since these grains are no longer a part of our diet, we need to be sure we replace the missing nutrients with other foods to avoid nutritional deficiencies.

Celiac disease destroys the villi of the small intestine, decreasing their ability to absorb nutritional substances such as fats, carbohydrates, protein, vitamins and minerals. The inflammation and damage to the intestinal villi result in the malabsorption of essential vitamins, minerals, and calories. We aren't getting the nutrition we need to stay healthy and we increase the risk for other diseases. Anemia is common among individuals with Celiac disease. Low levels of Vitamin B12, Vitamin B9 (Folate) and Vitamin B2 (Riboflavin) can result in anemia. Iron deficiency is also associated with anemia and is a typical result of inflammation of the small intestine. Malabsorption can cause deficiencies in other vitamins and minerals such as iron, calcium and Vitamin D. Diarrhea and fatty stools can cause low levels of magnesium, calcium and Vitamins A, D, E and K. Individuals with celiac disease also have decreased calcium and vitamin D absorption due to poor nutrient absorption. They may need to increase their intake of Vitamin D, calcium and Vitamin K to improve bone health and prevent osteopenia and/or osteoporosis. Osteopenia refers to bone mineral density (BMD) that is lower than normal but not low enough to be classified as osteoporosis.

Celiacs and those with Gluten-Sensitivity can't eat wheat, rye or barley. But what are we losing by removing those grains from our diet? We can replace wheat flour with other gluten-free flours and be ok, right? Not necessarily. We're not just removing bread from our diet. We're removing all the foods that contain wheat, rye and barley. All the meats with a bread coating, the hamburgers and chicken sandwiches that are served on wheat buns at all those fast food restaurants, the take-out pizza. We can't eat regular pasta at home or in a restaurant. Most salads are served with croutons made from wheat bread. I used to stop at the bakery for fresh rolls and donuts when I could still eat gluten, so the baked goods are out now, too. I'm not trying to make you sad by telling you all the foods you can't have anymore. I'm just trying to point out how many of our foods contain wheat. Even if you never ate a slice of bread, most of your food was coated, filled or served on wheat. This is why you need to be sure to replace the vitamins and other nutrients found in wheat, rye and barley with other foods that have the same nutrients. If you don't, you are at risk for deficiencies.

So, exactly what nutrients are in wheat, rye and barley. You might be surprised at how much nutrition is packed in those tiny kernels:

Wheat contains Iron, Zinc, Selenium, Magnesium and Vitamins B1 (Thiamine), B2 (Riboflavin) and B3 (Niacin).

Rye contains Protein, Potassium, Zinc, Calcium, Iron, Magnesium and Vitamins A, Vitamins B1 (Thiamine), B2 (Riboflavin) and B3 (Niacin), B5 (Pantothenic Acid), B6 (Pyridoxine) and B9 (Folate) as well as Vitamin E and K.

Barley contains Calcium, Iron, Protein, Potassium Zinc and Vitamins B1 (Thiamine), B2 (Riboflavin) and B3 (Niacin), B5 (Pantothenic Acid), B6 (Pyridoxine) and B9 (Folate) and Vitamin E.

These three little grains are packed with a lot of nutrition!

The question now is how do I replace all those vitamins and minerals? What foods should I eat? Listed below are the vitamins and minerals that can become deficient with Celiac disease, the purpose of each nutrient and alternate foods that contain the vital nutrients. This will help you decide how to eat a balanced diet.

Iron
Iron is necessary to help red blood cells deliver oxygen to the rest of our body and helps our bodies fight off infections. Vitamin C helps the body absorb iron.

Deficiency can cause irritability, tiredness, dizziness, inability to concentrate, depression, hair loss and brittle nails.

<u>Foods high in iron</u>
Beef
Poultry
Fish and Oysters
Beans & Lentils
Nuts and Peanuts
Molasses
Potatoes
Broccoli
Asparagus
Artichokes
Eggs
Tofu
Dried apricots, dates & raisins.

Vitamin D
Vitamin D is required for bone development, neuromuscular function, a healthy immune system, control of inflammation, cell growth and to help with the absorption of calcium.

Deficiency can lead to osteopenia and osteoporosis as well as depression, fatigue and heart disease.

Foods high in Vitamin D
Herring, catfish, herring, salmon, trout, halibut
Shrimp & oysters
Orange juice
Mushrooms
Yogurt
Salami, ham & sausage
Eggs

Calcium

Calcium keeps your muscles and nerves working properly. Calcium is needed for strong bones, helps your blood clot and is good for your heart.

Deficiency can be vague, take years to develop, and may not be noticeable until osteopenia or osteoporosis have developed. Warning signals can be back or neck pain, bone tenderness, stooped posture (abnormal curving of the spine and humpback)

Foods high in calcium
Cheese and milk
Sesame Seeds
Tofu
Almonds & brazil nuts
Flax seeds (flax seed oil has no calcium)
Yogurt & ice cream
Green, leafy vegetables
Herring
Dried herbs – thyme, dill, marjoram, sage, rosemary, oregano, spearmint, parsley, poppy seed, basil

Magnesium

Magnesium is essential for muscle and nerve function, a healthy immune system, maintaining heart rhythm and building strong bones. Magnesium is also needed for proper calcium absorption.

Deficiencies can result in muscle weakness and fatigue, memory problems, hyperexcitability, anxiety, restless leg syndrome (RLS), inability to sleep, nausea and vomiting.

<u>Foods high in magnesium</u>
Rice bran
Squash, pumpkin and watermelon seeds
Dark chocolate
Cocoa powder
Flax seeds
Sesame seeds, sunflower seeds, pine nuts
Almonds, cashews & brazil nuts
Molasses
Soybeans

Vitamin A
Vitamin A is necessary for good eyesight, boosting the immune system, healthy skin and to help your body fight off viral infections.

Deficiencies can lead to numerous viral infections, night blindness and bumpy skin.

<u>Foods high in Vitamin A</u>
Liver
Sweet potatoes
Carrots
Dark, leafy greens
Butternut squash
Dried apricots
Cantaloupe
Dried herbs – parsley, basil, marjoram, oregano
Paprika, red pepper, cayenne, chili powder

Vitamin E
Vitamin E helps can help to protect against heart disease, cancer and age-related eye damage (macular degeneration). It helps to

promote healing and helps to keep skin hydrated. It is crucial for forming red blood cells.

Deficiencies can cause neurological problems due to poor nerve conduction. Weakness and drooping upper eyelid, enlarged prostate and miscarriage.

<u>Foods high in Vitamin E</u>
Sunflower seeds
Almonds, pine nuts, peanuts
Dried apricots
Green olives
Spinach
Taro root
Paprika, red chili powder
Dried basil & oregano

Vitamin K

Vitamin K is required for proper blood clotting. The "K" is derived from the German word "koagulation" which refers to the process of blood clot formation. The body stores very little Vitamin K and needs to be replenished through dietary means.

Deficiencies include unexplained or easy bruising or bleeding, frequent nose bleeds, bleeding gums, blood in the urine and/or stools and heavy menstrual bleeding. Studies have determined a link between low Vitamin K levels and osteoporosis.

<u>Foods high in Vitamin K</u>
Dark, leafy greens
Green onions (scallions)
Brussels Sprouts
Broccoli
Chili powder, curry, paprika, cayenne
Dried herbs – basil, sage, thyme, parsley, coriander, marjoram, oregano
Asparagus
Cabbage

Cucumber pickles
Prunes

7 "B" Vitamins

The 8 B vitamins help the body convert food (carbohydrates) into fuel (glucose), which is used to produce energy. They are needed for healthy skin, eyes, hair and liver. B vitamins help the nervous system function properly and are necessary for brain function. The body does not store B vitamins, so they must be replenished by the foods we eat.

Vitamin B1 (Thiamin)

Thiamine helps to strengthen the immune system and improves the body's ability to endure stressful conditions.

Deficiencies include fatigue, irritability, depression, abdominal cramping, loss of mental alertness, difficulty breathing and heart damage.

Foods high in Vitamin B1 (Thiamin)
Pork
Organ meats (liver, kidneys)
Rice
Beans and legumes
Molasses
Sesame seeds and sesame butter
Sunflower seeds
Pine nuts
Pistachio nuts, Macadamia nuts, Pecans
Fish
Dried herbs – coriander, poppy seeds, sage, paprika, mustard seed, rosemary & thyme

Vitamin B2 (Riboflavin)
Riboflavin fights damaging particles in the body known as free radicals. Free radicals damage cells and DNA in addition to leading

to heart disease and cancer. Vitamin B2 is needed for growth and red blood cell production. It is also needed for normal vision and may help prevent cataracts.

Deficiencies include stunted growth, fatigue, digestive problems, cracks and sores in the corners of the mouth, swollen tongue, sensitivity to light and sore, swollen throat.

Foods high in Vitamin B2 (Riboflavin):
Organ meats (liver, kidneys)
Wild rice
Mushrooms
Soybeans
Milk products & yogurt
Eggs
Broccoli
Brussels sprouts
Spinach
Dried herbs – paprika, chili powder, coriander, spearmint, parsley
Dried ancho chilies
Sun-dried tomatoes
Sesame Seeds

Vitamin B3 (Niacin)
Niacin helps to improve circulation and boosts your "good" cholesterol. It is needed for DNA repair. It helps our bodies absorb calcium.

Deficiencies include:
Fatigue
Cold sores
Vomiting
Depression
Cracked, scaly skin
Diarrhea
Memory loss
Dermatitis (skin rash)

Foods high in Niacin:
Rice bran
Fish (Tuna, anchovies, swordfish)
Liver
Peanuts
Veal
Chicken
Bacon
Sun-dried Tomatoes
Paprika

Vitamin B5 (Pantothenic Acid)

Vitamin B5 helps the body break down fats & carbohydrates for energy. It is critical in the manufacture of red blood cells and plays an important part in maintaining a healthy digestive tract. Pantothenic Acid is used by the body to synthesize cholesterol.

Deficiencies:
Fatigue
Insomnia
Depression
Irritability
Vomiting
Abdominal pain
Burning feet
Upper respiratory infections

Foods high in Vitamin B5 (Pantothenic Acid)
Liver
Rice ban
Sunflower seeds
Whey powder (if not lactose intolerant)
Mushrooms
Cheese
Sun-dried tomatoes
Fish

Vitamin B6 (Pyridoxine)

Vitamin B6 breaks down proteins, keeps blood sugar levels within normal range and maintain normal nerve function. It helps your body make antibodies and make hemoglobin. Hemoglobin carries oxygen in the red blood cells to the tissues. A deficiency in Vitamin B6 can cause anemia. Pyridoxine helps to improve the immune system.

Deficiencies:
Confusion
Depression
Irritability
Mouth and tongue sores
Skin problems
Weakened immune system

Foods high in Vitamin B6 (Pyridoxine):
Rice bran
Dried herbs – chili powder, paprika, garlic powder, tarragon, sage, spearmint, bail, chives, bay leaves, rosemary, dill, onion powder, oregano, marjoram
Pistachios
Raw garlic
Liver
Fish
Sunflower and Sesame seeds
Pork (lean)
Molasses and sorghum syrup (sorghum flour)
Hazelnuts (Filberts)

Vitamin B9 (Folic Acid)

Folic acid is important for proper brain function and plays a vital role in mental and emotional health. It works with Vitamin B12 to make red blood cells and helps the body utilize iron.

Deficiencies:

Stunted growth
Loss of appetite
Shortness of breath
Diarrhea
Memory problems
Mental sluggishness
Mouth and tongue swelling
Irritability

Foods high in Vitamin B6 (Folic Acid)
Liver
Sunflower seeds
Dried herbs – spearmint, rosemary, basil, coriander, marjoram, thyme, bay leaf, parsley
Soybeans
Spinach
Dark leafy greens
Bean sprouts (soybean and pea sprouts)
Beans (Pinto, Garbanzo, black beans, lima beans, navy beans)
Asparagus
Peanuts

Vitamin B12 (Cobalamin)

Vitamin B12 helps in the production of red blood cells and keeps nerve cells healthy. It helps your cells metabolize protein, carbohydrates and fat.

Deficiencies:

Tingling or numbness of feet
Heart palpitations
Depression
Memory problems
B12 anemia
Weakness, light-headedness
Pale skin

Easy bruising or bleeding (nose bleeds, bleeding gums)
Diarrhea
Constipation
Difficulty walking

Foods high in Vitamin B12 (Cobalamin)
Liver
Clams, Oysters & Octopus
Fish
Crab & Lobster
Beef
Lamb
Cheese
Eggs

People with celiac disease also have decreased calcium and vitamin D absorption and may need calcium, vitamin D, and vitamin K supplements to improve bone health and prevent osteopenia or osteoporosis. This is particularly true of children and teens who have a lower bone mineral density than typical children and may be at greater risk of bone fractures.

Osteoporosis refers to very low bone mineral density. Osteopenia refers to bone mineral density (BMD) that is lower than normal peak BMD but not low enough to be classified as osteoporosis.

THE TRUTH ABOUT MSG & GLUTEN

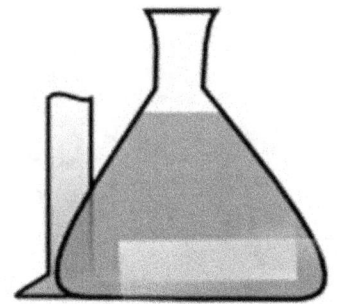

The Truth About MSG & Gluten

There is much controversy about MSG and gluten. Does MSG contain gluten or not? Simply put – not today, in the US.

First, what IS MSG?

Monosodium Glutamate (MSG) "is obtained by the fermentation of carbohydrates and by using bacteria or yeast" (Wikipedia). In 1907 Kikunae Ikeda isolated MSG from seaweed extract to be used as a flavor enhancer. In 1909 MSG was patented by Ajinomoto Corp. From 1909 to the mid-1960's, MSG was produced by the hydrolysis of wheat gluten. Today, it is produced in the US by the fermentation of starch, sugar beets, sugar cane or molasses. Many times "hydrolyzed proteins" are used by the food industry to enhance flavor. "A hydrolyzed protein is any protein that has been chemically broken down into amino acids. Hydrolyzed protein contains free amino acids, such as glutamate." " This chemical breakdown of proteins results in the formation of free glutamate which joins with free sodium to form MSG" (Wikipedia)

MSG, also known as sodium glutamate, is "a sodium salt of the naturally occurring non-essential amino acid glutamic acid." (Wikipedia) Glutamic acid is an amino acid that leads to the formation of glutamate. Glutamate is found in all living things such as meat, dairy, eggs, legumes (beans & peas) and seaweed. It helps remove nitrogen from the body and is a key molecule in cellular metabolism.

However, it is also "the most abundant excitatory neurotransmitter in the vertebrate nervous system and is involved in cognitive functions like learning and memory in the brain." (Wikipedia)

So to sum things up, MSG does not contain gluten, if manufactured in the US today.

Can Celiacs and those with gluten sensitivities eat MSG?

It does not contain gluten if manufactured in the US. Some Celiacs have reactions to MSG, some do not. Trial and error and experience will help you make a choice about your ability to eat MSG.

Is MSG safe to eat?

MSG is an ingredient in many manufactured foods and it is possible to consume high doses of MSG over a short period of time. Many people are sensitive to MSG and can have reactions similar to the reactions of people who have Celiac disease or gluten sensitivity.

Symptoms of MSG Toxicity can include:

Mouth lesions, migraines, diarrhea, vomiting, Asthma symptoms, chest pain, cough, gagging reflex, hives, blisters, numbness of face and extremities, cotton mouth, dark circles under eyes, constipation, urinary problems, swelling of prostate, acid reflux, gall bladder problems, restless leg syndrome, ear problems, loss of memory, seizures, balance issues, behavioral problems, ADHD, joint pain, TMJ, numbness or paralysis, Anaphylactic Shock . . . . . the list goes on. You decide if MSG is safe for you to eat, whether you have issues with gluten or not.

As always, it is up to the individual to decide if a product is safe for them to eat or not.

CHILDREN & SCHOOLS

504 PLAN

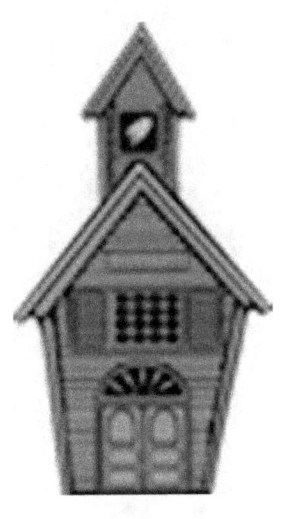

Children and Schools – 504 Plan

If you have a school-age child who needs to follow a gluten-free lifestyle, you may want to consider initiating a 504 Plan at their school. The 504 Plan is a Federal civil rights statute that was designed to protect the rights of individuals with disabilities in programs and activities that receive federal funds from the US Department of Education. Any child with a disability that significantly impacts a major life activity is protected by this law. This law has determined that Celiac disease is a disability because it affects a major life function – eating. This statute applies to all children with all types of disabilities. Each school may have their own interpretation of what the 504 Plan covers.

The law requires that school districts must offer gluten-free meals at no extra cost. It does not educate the schools on what is considered a gluten-free meal, nor does it educate them about the dangers of cross-contamination. Parents must take the initiative to put a 504 Plan into action and must be responsible for educating the school. Education is the key to keeping your child safe and healthy. You can't be with your child 24 hours a day, 7 days a week – you must depend on others to be informed about what will make your child sick. They must be willing to strictly follow the gluten-free requirements.

Celiac disease, itself, does not automatically qualify for a 504 Plan. Each person must make an individual argument for why the child should qualify for a 504 Plan and how detrimental to their education it would be if a 504 Plan was not accepted. Gluten-free lunches are not the only area that are affected. Your child's social, academic, emotional and physical concerns will also be affected because of their Celiac disease.

Contact your child's school and tell them you want to initiate a 504 Plan for your child and ask for the name of the person to discuss this with. Request a Section 504 evaluation. Request that the meeting include the principal, school nurse, head cook, dietitian and your child's teacher.

Be prepared to explain what Celiac disease is, the reactions your child may experience if they eat foods that contain gluten and the importance of avoiding cross-contamination. If your child experiences headaches, diarrhea or "brain fog" let the school know so they can watch for these reactions. Describe how gluten-free foods need to be stored and prepared in a separate area from the rest of the food to avoid cross-contamination.

There is no standard "504 Plan" document that can just be filled in and given to the school. You and your child's school will need to create an individual 504 Plan specific to your child.

There are areas in the school, in addition to the lunchroom, where there is a chance of gluten contamination.

Cafeteria requirements:

a. The table your child eats at must be washed with soap and water before they sit down to eat, to be sure there is no gluten on the table from previous use.

b. Your child's gluten-free food needs to be stored separate from foods that contain gluten

c. Your child's food needs to be prepared separately from foods that contain gluten. This includes separate pans, utensils and countertops.

d. The person preparing the food needs to wash their hands and use new rubber gloves before handling your child's gluten-free food, to be sure there is no gluten on their hands from handling foods that contain gluten.

e. List who is responsible for preparing and handling your child's food. Have the school write out what safeguards will be in place to assure that your child only receives gluten-free foods.

f. Include a list of acceptable foods that are gluten-free that can be provided – as long as they have been prepared in a separate area.

Classroom requirements:

a. No products containing gluten should be used by your child. To make the transition easier, you may want to offer to supply gluten-free finger paints, glue, paste, paints, crayons and markers for your child. These supplies need to be kept separate from the supplies the other students use and should be used only by your child.

b. Your child cannot share treats (birthdays, celebrations, etc.) brought in by other children, unless the teacher can verify that they are gluten-free. It would be helpful to supply the teacher with a list of acceptable gluten-free treats. You can also offer to leave a supply of gluten-free treats that your child can have when their classmates have treats that contain gluten. These treats need to be kept in a separate area and used only for your child.

c. Your child's teacher needs to be aware of the symptoms your child may experience if they are contaminated by gluten. If diarrhea is one of the effects of gluten that your child experiences, the teacher needs to be aware that your child is to be allowed to use the bathroom when necessary. Many classrooms allow only specific bathroom breaks. A reaction to gluten is an exception.

d. Classroom attendance may be affected when your child is contaminated by gluten. Many times "brain fog" is a result of gluten. If your child experiences "brain fog" their teacher should be aware of what signs to look for – inattentive, they forget what they were doing, short attention span, falling asleep at their desk, etc.

School Nurse

a. Explain to the school nurse what symptoms to be aware of, should your child accidentally eat a food that contains gluten, or if your child comes into contact with products that contain gluten.

b. Explain what steps the nurse should take at this time. (ie: call parent, give child pain reliever, let child rest, etc.)

School Counselor

a. Following a gluten-free lifestyle can be challenging at times, especially for children. In addition to learning to live gluten-free, they also deal with peer pressure and the desire to NOT be "different". Children must learn to cope with the emotions of Celiac disease. The school counselor needs to be aware of the "typical" emotions, the feeling s of grief and anger that your child may experience in learning to live gluten-free.

There is no "standard" 504 Plan. A 504 Plan is created for each child, particular to their requirements. Certain information should be detailed and included in your child's 504 Plan.

A 504 Plan needs to have specific instructions for everyone involved and should include the following sections:
:

Part 1: Student information

a. Student's name
b. Name of student's parents
c. Student's date of birth
d. Student's current grade
e. Name of current school district

Part 2: Initial 504 Plan meeting information

a. Name of child's parents
b. Name of current teacher(s)
c. Name of school nurse
d. Name of principal
e. Name of head cook or kitchen contact
f. Name of school counselor

Part 3: Background information

a. Explanation of Celiac disease or gluten sensitivity

b. Student's reactions to gluten that can be expected (ie: diarrhea, nausea, headache, brain fog, Dermatitis Herpetiformis, etc.)

c. Explanation of cross-contamination

d. Explanation of foods that could make your child sick

e. Explanation of gluten-free foods that are safe

f. Environmental contamination issues (ie: airborne gluten, paste, paints, gluten left on hands or tables from foods that contain gluten such as snacks, etc.)

g. Date of diagnosis

Part 4: Child's current condition overview

a. Parents should explain what cross-contamination is and the dangerous health issues gluten poses to your child

b. Explain that the major life activity affected by Celiac disease or gluten sensitivity is the child's food source

c. Parents should explain that foods is not the only item that may include gluten. Explain that personal care products (such as soaps, lotions, medications and bandaids) can contain gluten.

d. Provide a list of contact names and phone numbers to be contacted if gluten contamination is suspected.

Part 5 – Training for School Staff needed

a. Explain what precautions need to be taken in the classroom (ie: gluten-free crayons, glue, paint, etc. to be used ONLY for this child. These products are not to be shared by other classmates to avoid cross-contamination.)

b. Will the child be allowed additional bathroom breaks if needed?

c. Explain the information and training that will be given to other students in child's classroom

d. Explain what precautions need to be taken in the lunchroom and kitchen. (ie: preparation of gluten-free foods in separate area of kitchen, food preparers need to wash hands and wear new rubber gloves when handling gluten-free foods, etc.)

e. Explain where the child's lunch and snacks will be stored in order to avoid cross-contamination.

f. What gluten-free options will be available for the child when other children bring in treats for birthdays and holiday celebrations? Who will provide these gluten-free options? Where will these gluten-free options be stored?

g. Explain what precautions need to be taken by school nurse. (ie: what medications should be dispensed to student, brand names of safe GF medications. If parents will provide gluten-free medications such as pain relievers, allergy medication, acidophilus, etc., determine where these gluten-free products will be stored and who will have access to them. They need to be kept ONLY for student and never shared with other students.)

h. Explain who will provide training for school staff – parents need to be closely involved in training.

i. Instructions on how to read an ingredient list and how to recognize other names for gluten. Parents should provide a list of "other names for gluten" to school.

Part 5 – Documents to support the need for a 504 Plan

a. IHP - Individualized Health Care Plan
"The National Associate of School Nurses has determined that any student with a relatively complex health condition, or a need for modification of the school environment due to a health condition, should have an IHP. They have also determined that the school nurse should be responsible for writing the IHP in collaboration with the student, the student's parents and the student's physician."

An IHP helps to ensure that all necessary information, needs and plans are considered to maximize the student's participation and performance in school. The IHP also covers other aspects of care such as a student's knowledge about their condition, self-care abilities and any modifications needed to enhance learning and prevent emergencies

b. A letter from your child's doctor stating:

1. That your child has been diagnosed with Celiac disease or gluten sensitivity

2. How your child's restricted diet affects a major life activity – eating

3. A list of the foods that must be omitted from their diet – wheat, rye, barley and oats

4. The doctor should explain that gluten-free food is necessary to keep your child healthy. He should also explain that this restriction does not apply just to food. Your child needs to avoid products that contain gluten such as Play Doh, paints, fingerpaints, bandaids, lotions, soaps, glue and paste.

c. An Emergency Health Care Plan

1. What are your child's signs and symptoms of gluten cross-contamination?

2. What are your child's signs and symptoms of full gluten contamination?

3. What are the signs and symptoms of a gluten contact reaction?

4. Outline the steps to be taken when your child is contaminated by gluten. Who should be involved (ie: teacher, school nurse, kitchen coordinator, etc.)

5. Explain when school personnel can handle a gluten situation and what medications, if any, should be administered. Explain the amount of medication to be administered.

6. Explain when parents should be called.

7. Determine if child should remain in class or be taken to nurse's office.

8. Does your child wear a medical alert bracelet or necklace?

Part 6 – Additional information

1. Specify how often the 504 Plan will be reviewed. (example: "This 504 Plan shall be reviewed and amended at the

beginning of each school year or more often if deemed necessary by parents, teachers or school nurse.")

2. Specify who can request a 504 plan review.

3. Specify where copies of the 504 Plan will be kept. (One copy should be kept in the school nurse's office, one copy in the child's classroom and one copy for the child's parents.)

4. A Self-Care Assessment Data Sheet should be kept with the 504 Plan at all locations. A Self-Care Assessment Data Sheet explains to what extent the child is responsible for managing their Celiac disease or gluten sensitivity. This Data Sheet could include information such as:

a. The child is able to read an ingredient list and is aware of which ingredients to avoid

b. The child is able to recognize foods that contain gluten (ie: wheat bread, baked goods with wheat ingredients, specific brand names of gluten products, etc.)

c. The child is able to recognize signs and symptoms of gluten contamination.

d. The child is able to verbally communicate above symptoms.

e. The child knows they must wash their hands after using a product that may contain gluten

f. The child knows they must was tables and desks before eating gluten-free foods

g. The child knows not to share food or eat food offered by another child or adult

h. The child knows to check with teachers and other adults to make sure their food does not contain gluten.

i. The child is knowledgeable of cross-contamination and is aware of the dangers of cross-contamination

j. The student knows what steps to take when they suspect they have been contaminated by gluten.

The 504 Plan should be signed by the Parents, child's Teacher, School Nurse, Lunchroom coordinator and child's Doctor.

It is important that your child's school is educated about Celiac disease, cross-contamination and the reactions that result from being contaminated with gluten. It is also important to educate your child. Ultimately, they are responsible for keeping themselves safe and healthy. They need to know what foods are safe, how to read an ingredient list, how to wash their hands after handling items that may contain gluten, how to ask questions about products they are going to use and what reactions to be aware of.

SOCIAL SITUATIONS AND EATING OUT

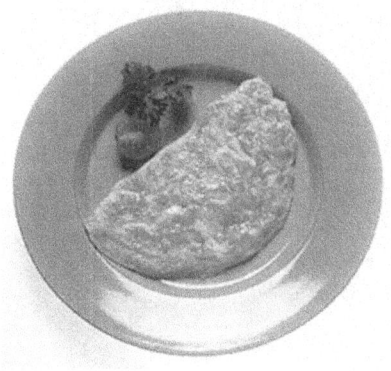

Social Situations & Eating Out

You can control the foods you eat and the chance of cross-contamination in your home because you can choose which foods are allowed in your home, where they are stored and who has access to the gluten-free foods. It can be much more challenging in social situations such as family gatherings, holidays and eating at someone else's home. Children want to spend time with their friends at play dates, sleepovers and birthday parties. In these situations you can't control which foods are available, whether they contain gluten or who handles the foods. There are so many opportunities for cross-contamination.

What do you do? How do you protect your child? How do you guarantee the food is safe?

First of all, nothing in life is guaranteed. Mistakes will be made, accidents will happen and there will be times that you and/or your child may become sick. When this happens, accept it, deal with the reactions and move forward.

Family Gatherings/Holidays

Family gatherings and holidays usually include food. Lots and lots of food. Many of these foods have ingredients that contain gluten, or may be cross-contaminated with gluten in the preparation. You can't control how others prepare their food. You can't insist that all the food served in these situations be gluten-free. How do you attend these gatherings and still avoid becoming sick from gluten? You can prepare for these situations by following a few easy steps:

1. Talk to the person who will be hosting the gathering. Ask what foods will be served. Will there be naturally gluten-free foods

such as fresh fruits and vegetables? Discuss the food preparation, the ingredients that will be used and the method of preparation.

2. Hosting a gathering takes a lot of preparation and work. People who don't deal with living gluten-free on a daily basis may not understand which ingredients are safe, or be aware of how cross-contamination can happen. Offer to bring your own gluten-free foods and store them separately. Bringing your own food allows you to enjoy spending time with the relatives and still be a part of the food celebration.

3. Some foods are naturally gluten-free, such as fresh fruits and vegetables and meat. Remember though, these naturally gluten-free foods can be contaminated during preparation and serving. A gluten-free vegetable dip can be contaminated by someone dipping a cracker into it, or by using a serving spoon that was used in a food that contains gluten. Set aside an individual serving of these foods before they are put on the table for others. Meat is gluten-free, but can be contaminated during preparation. Turkey that has been filled with wheat bread stuffing is no longer gluten-free. Meats with gravy made with wheat flour are no longer gluten-free.

4. Remember the main reason for these gatherings is to spend time with your family. The food is just a small part. Don't make food the main focus.

Social Gatherings

Joining friends at their homes for dinner, parties and eating in restaurants can be challenging, to say the least. There is no reason you need to avoid these situations, if you prepare for them in advance.

1. If you are meeting at a friend's house, call the person hosting the dinner and ask what foods will be served. Ask if any of the foods could be adjusted to be gluten-free. Offer to bring part of the meal, making sure your offering is gluten-free.

2. Attending parties, especially those that offer buffet items, can be more of a challenge. Again, you can call the host ahead of time and offer to bring a gluten-free choice or two to add to the buffet. Eating at home before the party is another option. Most social gatherings are more about spending time with the people, than eating food. Enjoy the time spent with friends.

3. Eating at a restaurant is a situation that offers the highest possibility of becoming "glutenized". Many restaurants now offer gluten-free items. The foods themselves don't contain gluten, but many of these same restaurants don't understand the cross-contamination issues. Management may understand the importance of gluten-free food preparation, but if they don't train their staff properly, there is always a chance for error or misunderstanding.

Call the restaurant ahead of time and ask if they offer gluten-free foods. Ask how the gluten-free food it prepared. Is it prepared in a separate area of the kitchen? Are separate pans and utensils used on the gluten-free food? Has the kitchen staff been trained in avoiding cross-contamination? Do they wash their hands or change their gloves before touching any gluten-free foods? Don't be afraid to ask detailed questions. Your health is at stake and you need to know how extensive their knowledge of gluten-free foods is.

Most gatherings are more about spending time with friends and family, than they are about eating food. If you focus more on the food that is available to you, than on the reason you're all getting together, you will miss the most important part of the gathering – the people.

IMMUNIZATIONS

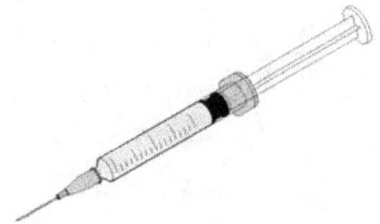

Immunizations

Many children with Celiac disease or a gluten sensitivity also have food allergies. The top 8 food allergens that must be listed on ingredient lists are wheat, corn, soy, eggs, dairy, peanuts, nuts and shellfish.

Immunizations, however, do not need to list any possible allergens. We are told that we need to have our children immunized against many diseases. Diseases that can cause dangerous health complications, possibly death. We are told that immunizations are safe for our children, but we are not told what is IN those immunizations. For many children, these immunizations ARE safe. But, for children who have allergies to one or more ingredient in the immunizations, they are NOT safe.

I originally researched the standard childhood immunizations to find out if any of them contained gluten. I am happy to report that I have yet to find an immunization by any of the manufacturers that contains gluten. I could have ended this chapter right here and told you there is no gluten in any immunization. But, gluten is not the only ingredient a parent needs to be concerned with. Celiac disease or gluten sensitivity is not the only health issue a parent needs to be concerned with.

My youngest granddaughter has Celiac disease. She also has an allergy to casein. When her mother and I read ingredient lists we need to be concerned with any gluten ingredients AND any dairy ingredients. Some children may have other food allergies in addition to Celiac disease. Some immunizations contain dairy or egg, some contain latex, formaldehyde, antibiotics and Aspartame. Depending on your child's reaction to these allergens, receiving an immunization that contains an ingredient that your child is allergic to could become life-threatening. Some of the immunizations contain Thimerosal. There is a great deal of controversy over whether or not this mercury-containing ingredient causes Autism. I could give you my own opinion, here, but it is up to every parent to make a personal choice for their child. Research and knowledge is the key to making an informed choice. A few very good websites to learn more about Thimerosal are:

www.generationrescue.org
www.autismspeaks.org
www.autism.com
www.nationalautismassociation.org/thimerosal.php

There are many companies that manufacture the same immunizations and each company uses their own ingredients in their immunizations. One may contain an ingredient that will make your child very sick, one may not. In order to make informed choices, as parents, you need to be aware of what your pediatrician is injecting into your child. It is up to each parent to decide if a particular immunization or an ingredient is safe for their child. In order to make an informed decision, you need information. On the following pages is a list of the most common childhood immunizations, the age schedule for each and specific manufacturer ingredients. This list does not contain every single manufacturer, just the most commonly used.

If your child has allergies or reactions to specific ingredients, you should ask your child's pediatrician for specific details on the immunizations he plans to give your child. Who is the manufacturer? What are the ingredients? If the pediatrician is unsure of the ingredients, ask for the manufacturers name and call them to ask about ingredients. At what age is this immunization safe to administer? Can the immunization be delayed until the child is older? What other health issues does your child have at the time they receive the immunization? Again, information is the key to making an informed decision regarding your child.

Immunizations

Vaccine	Ingredients	Ingredient Description	Manufacturrer
Recombivax			Merck & Co., Inc.
birth, 1 mo, 6 mo	Aluminum hydroxide	Antacid	800-672-6372
	Hepatitis B virus		
	GMO yeast		
	Thimerosal	mercury containing compound	

Vaccine	Ingredients	Ingredient Description	Manufacturrer
HBV and Hib conjugate vaccine	Aluminum hydroxide	Antacid	Merck & Co., Inc.
2 mo, 4 mo, 6 mo	**Formaldehyde**	colorless, flammable gas - known carcinogen	800-672-6372
booster at 12-15 mo	Yeast		
	Haemophilus influenzae B		
	Sodium borate	common roach killer, cleaner-Borax	
	Amino acids		
	Dextrose	sugar derived from corn *possible allergen*	
	Neisseria meningtides OMPC	protein carrier	
	Mineral salts		
	Nicotinamide adenine dinudleotide	coenzyme	
	Hemin chloride	ferric iron & chloride	
	Soy peptone	obtained from defatted soybean flour *possible allergen*	

Vaccine	Ingredients	Ingredient Description	Manufacturrer
Energi-B Recombinant	Aluminum hydroixide	Antacid	GlaxoSmithKline
birth, 1 mo, 6 mo	Thimerosal	mercury containing compound	800-366-8900
	Yeast		
	Sodium chloride	salt	
	Hepatitis B virus		
	Disodium phosphate dehydrate	sodium salt of phosphoric acid	
	Sodium dihydrogen phosphate dehydrate	laxative and Ph buffer	

Vaccine	Ingredients	Ingredient Description	Manufacturrer
Fendri-Hepatitis B (rDNA) vaccine	Yeast		GlaxoSmithKline
birth, 1 mo, 2 mo, 6 mo	Sodium chloride	salt	800-366-8900
	Aluminum phosphate	phospooric acid & aluminum salt	
	Hepatitis B virus		
	AsO4	stimulates immune system	

Vaccine	Ingredients	Ingredient Description	Manufacturrer
Recombivax HB (Hepatitis B)			
Vaccine	Aluminum hydroide	Antacid	Merck & Co., Inc.
birth, 1 mo, 6 mo	Hepatitis B virus		800-672-6372

Vaccine	Ingredients	Ingredient Description	Manufacturrer
Heavac (DTaP, IPV, HBV, Hib-Diptheria, tetanus, acellular pertussis, inactivated poliomyelitis, hepatitis B and Haemophilus influenzae type b conjugate vaccine)			Aventis Pasteur MSD
once at 2-12 months	Aluminum hydroxide	Antacid	800.VACCINE
booster 12-18 months	**Formaldehyde**	colorless, flammable gas - known carcinogen	
	Sucrose	sugar	
	Pertussis toxin		
	Filamentos hemagglutinin	a protein of pertussin	
	Diptheria toxoid		
	Tetanus toxoid		
	Bovine (cow) serum	blood plasma from cow	
	Sodium hydroide	lye	
	Hepatitis B virus		
	Medium 199	a complex medium of amino acids, mineral salts, vitamins, polysorbate 80 and other substances diluted in water	

143

Vaccine	Ingredients	Ingredient Description	Manufacturrer
Infanrix Penta	Aluminum hydroxide	Antacid	GlaxoSmithKline
2 mo, 3 mo, 4 mo, 11 mo	2-Phenoyethanol	preservative	800-366-8900
	Pertussis toxin		
	Filamentos hemagglutinin	a protein of pertussis	
	Pertactin	bacteria that causes pertussis	
	aluminum phosphate	phosphoric acid & aluminum salt	
	Diptheria toxoid		
	Tetanus toxoid		
	Hepatitis B virus		
	Polio virus		
	Medium 199	a complex medium of amino acids, mineral salts, vitamins, polysorbate 80 and other substances diluted in water	

Vaccine	Ingredients	Ingredient Description	Manufacturrer
Shanvac-B	Aluminum hydroxide	Antacid	Shantha Biotechnics
Hepatitis B vaccine IP (r-DNA)	Thimerosal	mercury containing compound	Pvt. Ltd.
birth, 1 mo, 2 mo, booster 12 mo	Hepatitis B virus		

Vaccine	Ingredients	Ingredient Description	Manufacturrer
Pediarix	Aluminum hydroxide	Antacid	GlaxoSmithKline
injections from 6 wks to 7 yrs	**Formaldehyde**	**colorless, flammable gas - known carcinogen**	800-366-8900
	Neomycin	**antibiotic**	
	Polymyxin B	**antiobiotic**	
	Polysorbate 80	surfactant (reduces surface tension) and emulsifier (blends substances)	
	Thimerosal	**mercury containing compoun**	
	Yeast		
	Pertussis toxin		
	Filamentos hemagglutinin	a protein of pertussis	
	Pertactin	bacteria that causes pertusis	
	Tetanus toxoid		
	Sodium chloride	salt	
	Polio virus		
	* Stopper vial may contain dry latex rubber *	***possible allergen***	

Vaccine	Ingredients	Ingredient Description	Manufacturrer
Pediarix	Aluminum hydroxide	Antacid	GlaxoSmithKline
injections from 6 wks to 7 yrs	**Formaldehyde**	**colorless, flammable gas - known carcinogen**	800-366-8900
	Neomycin	**antibiotic**	
	Polymyxin B	**antiobiotic**	
	Polysorbate 80	surfactant (reduces surface tension) and emulsifier (blends substances)	
	Thimerosal	**mercury containing compoun**	
	Yeast		
	Pertussis toxin		
	Filamentos hemagglutinin	a protein of pertussis	
	Pertactin	bacteria that causes pertusis	
	Tetanus toxoid		
	Sodium chloride	salt	
	Polio virus		
	*** Stopper vial may contain dry latex rubber ***	***possible allergen***	

Vaccine	Ingredients	Ingredient Description	Manufacturrer
DT-Polio	**Formaldehyde**	colorless, flammable gas - known carcinogen	Sanofi Pasteur
2 mo, 4 mo, 6 mo, 18 mo,	**Neomycin**	antibiotic	800-822-2463
4-6 years	2-Phenoxyethanol	preservative	
	Polymyxin B	antibiotic	
	Aluminum phosphate	absorbs toxins	

Vaccine	Ingredients	Ingredient Description	Manufacturrer
Tritanrix HepB Diphtheria, tetanus, pertussis and hepatitis B	Yeast		GlaxoSmithKline
3 injections, 1 mo apart	Sodium Chloride	salt	800-366-8900
	Aluminum phosphate	phosphoric acid & aluminum salt	
	Diphtheria toxoid		
	Tetanus toxoid		
	Hepatitis B virus		
	Aluminum oide	used to produce aluminum metal	

Vaccine	Ingredients	Ingredient Description	Manufacturrer
Twinrix Junior Hepatitis A and Hepatitis B Vaccine	Formaldehyde	colorless, flammable gas - known carcinogen	GlaxoSmithKline
birth, 30 days, 12 mo	2-Phenoxyethanol	preservative	800-366-8900
	Thimerosal	mercury containing compound	
	Sodium chloride	salt	
	Hepatitis B virus		
	Polysorbate 20		
	Hepatitis A virus		
	Amino acids		
	Neomycin sulphate	antibiotic	

Vaccine	Ingredients	Ingredient Description	Manufacturer
RotaTeq (Prevention of Rotavirus Gastroenteritis)	Polysorbate 80	surfactant (reduces tension) and emulsifier (blends substances)	Merck & Co., Inc. 800-672-6372
	Sucrose	sugar	
2 mo, 4 mo, 6 mo	sodium phosphate-monobasic	sodium salt of phosphoric acid	
	Bovine (cow) serum	blood plasma from cow	
	sodium hydroxide	lye	
	Rotavirus (live)		
	Sodium citrate	sodium salt of citric acid	

Vaccine	Ingredients	Ingredient Description	Manufacturer
Certiva (DPAT) Diphtheria, Tetanus, Pertussis	Ammonium sulfate	Antacid	Baxter Healthcare 800-422-9837
	Aluminum hydroxide	Antacid	
2 mo, 4 mo, 6 mo, 15 mo	Formaldehyde	colorless, flammable gas - known carcinogen	
	Thimerosal	mercury contianing compound	
	Pertussis toxin		
	Diphtheria toxoid		
	Tetanum toxoid		
	Bovine (cow) serum	blood plasma from cow	
	Fetuin	blood proteins made in the liver	

Vaccine	Ingredients	Ingredient Description	Manufacturrer
Daptacel (DTaP)	Formaldehyde	colorless, flammable gas - known carcinogen	Sanofi Pasteur
2 mo, 4 mo, 6 mo, 17 mo	Glutaraldehyde	a hazardous chemical used to sterilize, contans a respiratory and skin sensitizer	800-822-2463
	Latex	*possible allergen*	
	2-Phenoxyethanol	preservative	
	Pertactin	bacteria that causes pertussis	
	Aluminum phosphate	absorbs toxins	
	Pertussis toxin		
	Diphtheria toxoid		
	Tetanus toxoid		

Vaccine	Ingredients	Ingredient Description	Manufacturrer
DTAP-IPV Poliomyelitis	Diphtheria toxoid		Statens Serum Institute
2 mo, 3 mo, 4 mo	Tetanus toxoid		+45-3268-3268
	Polio virus		
	Haemophilus influenzae B		

Vaccine	Ingredients	Ingredient Description	Manufacturrer
Heavac (Diphtheria, tetanus, acellular pertussis, inactivated poliomyelitis, hepatitis B, haemophilus influenzae type B) 2 - 12 mo, booster 12-18 mo	Aluminum hydroxide	Antacid	Aventis Pasteur MSD 800.VACCINE
	Formaldehyde	colorless, flammable gas - known carcinogen	
	Sucrose	sugar	
	Pertussis toxin		
	Filamentous hemagglutinin	protein that causes pertussis	
	Diphtheria toxoid		
	Tetanus toxoid		
	Bovine (cow) serum	blood plasma from cow	
	Sodium hydroxide	lye	
	Hepatitis B virus		
	Medium 199	a complex medium of amino acids, mineral salts, vitamins, polysorbate 80 and other substances diluted in water	
	Haemophilus influenzae B		
	Acetic acid	antibiotic	
	Trometamol	non-steroidal anti-inflammatory drug (NSAID)	
	Sodium Hydrogen carbonate	baking soda	
	Potassiumhydrogen phosphate	laxative & Ph buffer	
	Disodium hydrogen carbonate	sodium salt of phosphoric acid	

Vaccine	Ingredients	Ingredient Description	Manufacturrer
Infanrix Pental (Diphtheria, tetanus, acellusar, hepatitis B, inactivated polio)			
2 mo, 3 mo, 4 mo, 11 mo	Aluminum hydroxide	antacid	GlaxoSmithKline
	2-Phenoxyethanol	perservative	800-366-8900
	Pertussis toxin		
	Filamentous hemagglutinin	protein that causes pertussis	
	Pertactin	bacteria that causes pertussis	
	Aluminum phosphate	absorbs toxins	
	Diphtheria toxoid		
	Tetanus toxoid		
	Hepatitis B virus		
	Polio virus		
	Medium 199	a complex medium of amino acids, mineral salts, vitamins, polysorbate 80 and other substances diluted in water	

Vaccine	Ingredients	Ingredient Description	Manufacturrer
Peiari (HBV, DTaP, IPB and inactivated Polio)	Aluminum hydroxide	Antacid	GlaxoSmithKline
3 injections, 6 wks - 7yrs	Formaldehyde	colorless, flammable gas- known carcinogen	800-366-8900
	Neomycin	antibiotic	
	Polymyxin B	antibiotic	
	Polysorbate 80	surfactant (reduces surface tension) and emulsifier (blends substances)	
	Thimerosal	mercury containing compound	
	Yeast		
	Pertussis toxin		
	Filamentous hemagglutinin	protein that causes pertussis	
	Pertactin	bacteria that causes pertussis	
	Tetanus toxoid		
	Sodium chloride	salt	
	Polio virus		
	stopper vial may contain dry latex rubber	*possible allergen*	

Vaccine	Ingredients	Ingredient Description	Manufacturer
Quadracel (Diphtheria, tetanus, pertussis, absorbed with poliomyelitis)			Aventis Pasteur
2 mo, 4 mo, 6 mo, 18 mo	Formaldehyde	colorless, flammable gas - known carcinogen	800-VACCINE
	Neomycin	antibiotic	
	2-Phenoxyethanol	preservative	
	Polymyxin B	antibiotic	
	Polysorbate 80	surfactant (reduces surface tension) and emulsifier (blends substances)	
	Pertussis toxin		
	Filamentous hemagglutinin	protein that causes pertussis	
	Pertactin	bacteria that causes pertussis	
	Tetanus toxoid		
	Aluminum phosphate	absorbs toxins	
	Diphtheria toxoid		
	Bovine (cow) serum	blood plasma from cow	

Vaccine	Ingredients	Ingredient Description	Manufacturer
Tritanrix HB-HIB (Diphtheria, tetanus, pertussis, hepatitis B)			GlaxoSmithKline
1 injection - 6 weeks	Aluminum hydroxide	antacid	800-366-8900
	Yeast		
	Sodium chloride	salt	
	Aluminum phosphate	absorbs toxins	
	Diphtheria toxoid		
	Tetanus toxoid		
	Hepatitis B virus		

Vaccine	Ingredients	Ingredient Description	Manufacturrer
Repavax (Diphtheria, tetanus, pertussis, poliomyelitis)		colorless, flammable gas - known	Aventis Pasteur
booster after age 3	Formaldehyde	carcinogen	800-VACCINE
	Neomycin	antibiotic	
	2-Phenoxyethenol	preservative	
	Polymyxin B	antibiotic	
		surfactant (reduces surface tension)	
	Polysorbate 80	and emulsifier (blends substances)	
	Streptomycin	antibiotic	
	Pertussis toxin		
	Aluminum phosphate	absorbs toxins	
	Diphtheria toxoid		
	Tetanus toxoiod		
	Polio virus		
	Polyribosylribitol phosphate		
	Aluminum phosphate		
	African green monkey kidney cells		

Vaccine	Ingredients	Ingredient Description	Manufacturrer
Pnu-Imune 23	Thimerosal	mercury containing compound	Wyeth-Ayerst
single injection - 2 years	2-(ethylmercurithio) benzoic acid		800-934-5556
	Pleymococcal Polysaccharide		

Vaccine	Ingredients	Ingredient Description	Manufacturrer
Tritanrix HepB (Diphtheria, tetanum, pertussis (whole cell), hepatitis B			
	Thimerosal	mercury containing compound	GlaxoSmithKline
3 injections, 1 month apart	Yeast		800-366-8900
	Sodium chloride	salt	
	Aluminum phosphate	absorbs toxins	
	Diphtheria toxoid		
	Tetanus toxoid		
	Hepatitis B virus		
	Aluminum oxide	used to produce aluminum metal	

Vaccine	Ingredients	Ingredient Description	Manufacturrer
Prevnar	Latex	*possible allergen*	Wyeth-Ayerst
2 mo, 4 mo, 6 mo, 12 mo	Aluminum phosphate	absorbs toxins	800-934-5556
	soy protein	*possible allergen*	
	S. Pneumonia bacteria, inactivated		

Vaccine	Ingredients	Ingredient Description	Manufacturrer
Imova Polio	Formaldehyde	colorless, flammable gas - known carcinogen	Connaught Labs 800-822-2463
3 injections, 8 weeks apart	Neomycin	antibiotic	
booster 1 year later	Polymyxin B	antibiotic	
	Streptomycin	antibiotic	
	Bovine (cow) serum	blood plasma from cow	
	Polio virus		
	African green monkey kidney cells		
	Medium 199		

Vaccine	Ingredients	Ingredient Description	Manufacturrer
IPOL (Polio - inactivated)	Formaldehyde	colorless, flammable gas - known carcinogen	Sanofi Pasteur 800-822-2463
2 mo, 4 mo, 6 mo, 18 mo,	Neomycin	antibiotic	
4 - 6 years	2-Phenoyethanol	preservative	
	Polymyxin B	antibiotic	
	Streptomycin	antibiotic	
	Bovin (cow) serum	blood plasma from cow	
	Polio virus		
	*stopper vial may contain dry latex rubber	* possible allergen *	

156

Vaccine	Ingredients	Ingredient Description	Manufacturrer
Pediarix	Aluminum hydroxide	Antacid	GlaxoSmithKline
3 injections - 6 wks & 7 yrs	Formaldehyde	colorless, flammable gas - known carcinogen	800-366-8900
	Neomycin	antibiotic	
	Polymyxin B	antibiotic	
	Polysorbate 80	surfactant (reduces surface tension) and emulsifier (blends substances)	
	Thimerosal	mercury containing compound	
	Yeast		
	Pertussis toxin		
	Filamentous hemagglutinin	proten that causes pertussis	
	Pertactin	bacteria that causes pertussis	
	Tetanus toxoid		
	Sodium chloride	salt	
	Polio virus		
	*stopper vial may contan dry latex rubber	*possible allergen*	

Vaccine	Ingredients	Ingredient Description	Manufacturrer
Attenuvax (live measles virus vaccine)	Gelatin		Merck & Co., Inc.
12 mo, 4 yr	Neomycin	antibiotic	800-672-6372
	Sorbitol	sugar alcohol	
	sucrose	sugar	
	Sodium Chloride	salt	
	Bovine (cow) serum	blood plasma from cow	
	Sodium phosphate	sodium salt of phosphoric acid	
	Measles virus (live)		
	Egg protein	*possible allergen*	
	Human albumin	protein in human blood plasma	

Vaccine	Ingredients	Ingredient Description	Manufacturer
Diplovax HDC 4.0 (freeze-dried measles vaccine)	Gelatin		Biovax
9 mo, booster 18 mo	Humann diploid cells	batches of human cells grown in a lab	508-793-0001
	MRC5 proteins	batches of human cells grown in a lab	
	Sorbitol	sugar alcohol	
	Measles virus (live)		

Vaccine	Ingredients	Ingredient Description	Manufacturrer
M-M-Rvax (measles & mumps live virus)	Gelatin		Merck & Co., Inc.
12 mo	Neomycin	antibiotic	800-672-6372
	Sorbitol	sugar alcohol	
	Sodium chloride	salt	
	Bovine (cow)serum	blood plasma from cow	
	Sodium phosphate	sodium salt of phosphoric acid	
	Measles virus (live)		
	Mumps virus		
	Human albumin	protein in human blood plasma	

Vaccine	Ingredients	Ingredient Description	Manufacturrer
M-R VAX, M-R VA II	Gelatin		Merck & Co., Inc.
(measles & rubella live vaccine)	Human diploid cells	batches of human cells grown in a lab	800-672-6372
1 injection - 12 mo+	MRC5 proteins	batches of human cells grown in a lab	
	Neomycin	antibiotic	
	Sorbitol	sugar alcohol	
	Measles virus (live)		
	Rubella virus		
	Chick embryo cells	*possible allergen*	

Vaccine	Ingredients	Ingredient Description	Manufacturrer
M-M-RVAXPro (measles, mumps, rubella - live)	Gelatin		Merck & Co., Inc.
12 mo	Monosodium Glutamate (MSG)	*possible allergen*	800-672-6372
	Neomycin	antibiotic	
	Phenol	disinfectant	
	Sorbitol	sugar alcohol	
	Sodium bicarbonate	baking soda	
	Sucrose	sugar	
	Sodium phosphate	sodium salt of phosphoric acid	
	Sodium hydroxide	lye	
	Hydrochloride acid	corrosive mineral acid	
	Potassium phosphate	salt of potassium & phosphate	
	Measles virus (live)		
	Mumps viurs		
	Rubella virus		
	Minimum essential medium		
	Medium 199	a complex medium of amino acids, mineral salts, vitamins, polysorbate 80 and other substances diluted in water	

Vaccine	Ingredients	Ingredient Description	Manufacturrer
MMR II (measels, mumps, rubella - live vaccine)	Gelatin		Merck & Co., Inc.
1 injection - 12 mo+	**Neomycin**	Antibiotic	800-672-6372
	Sorbitol	sugar alcohol	
	Sucrose	sugar	
	Sodium chloride	salt	
	Bovine (cow) serum	blood plasma from cow	
	Sodium phosphate	sodium salt of phosphoric acid	
	Measles virus (live)		
	Mumps virus		
	Rubella virus		
	Egg protein		
	Human albumin	protein in human blood plasma	

Vaccine	Ingredients	Ingredient Description	Manufacturrer
Morbilvax (live measles)	Neomycin	antibiotic	Novartis
2 injections between 9-18 mo	Measles virus (live)		800-452-0051
	Chick embryo cells	*possible allergen*	
	Kanamycin	antibiotic	

161

Vaccine	Ingredients	Ingredient Description	Manufacturrer
Priori (measles, mumps, rubella - live)	Human diploid cells	batches of human cells grown in a lab	GlaxoSmithKline
12 mo, booster 4 yrs	MRC5 proteins	batches of human cells grown in a lab	800-366-8900
	Sorbitol	sugar alcohol	
	Measles virus (live)		
	Mumps virus		
	Rubella virus		
	Chick embryo cells	*possible allergen*	
	Lactose	*possible allergen*	
	Mannitol	sugar alcohol	
	Amino acids		
	Human albumin	protein in human blook plasma	
	Neomycin sulphate	antibiotic	

Vaccine	Ingredients	Ingredient Description	Manufacturrer
Trimovax	Measles virus (live)		Aventis
1 injection 12 mo	Mumps virus		800-VACCINE
1 injection 3-6 yrs	Rubella virus		
	Human albumin	protein in human blood plasma	

Vaccine	Ingredients	Ingredient Description	Manufacturrer
ACWY Vax (meningitis vaccine)	Lactose	*possible allergen*	GlaxoSmithKline
1 injection - 2 yrs & older	Meningococcalpolysaccharide s W135		800-366-8900

Vaccine	Ingredients	Ingredient Description	Manufacturrer
Meningitec	Latex	*possible allergen*	Wyeth-Ayerst
6 wks, 1 mo, 2 mo	Sodium chloride	salt	800-934-5556
	Aluminum phosphate	absorbs toxins	
	Bovine (cow) serum	blood plasma from cow	
	Meningococcal Group C oligosaccharide		
	Diphtheriaj CRM 197 protein		

Vaccine	Ingredients	Ingredient Description	Manufacturer
Varivax (chicken pox live virus)	Gelatin		Merck & Co., Inc.
2 injections	Monosodium glutamate (MSG)	*possible allergen*	800-672-6372
	Human diploid cells	batches of human cells grown in a lab	
	MRC5 proteins	batches of human cells grown in a lab	
	Neomycin	antibiotic	
	Sucrose	sugar	
	Sodium chloride	salt	
	Sodium phosphate monobasic	sodium salt of phosphoric acid	
	Sodium phosphate dibasic dodecahydrate	sodium salt of phosphoric acid	
	Bovine (cow) serum	blood plasma from cow	
	Potassium phosphate		
	Human diploid cells	batches of human cells grown in a lag	
	EDTA	stabilizing agent	
	Potassium phosphate	salts of potassium & phosphate	
	Glutamate	salts of glutamic acid	

WHAT ABOUT "The Other Side"

A STORY FROM A NON-CELIAC

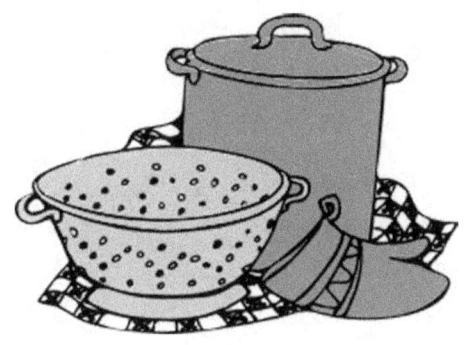

Living with a Celiac

Learning to live a gluten-free lifestyle can be challenging for Celiacs and those with a gluten sensitivity. There are numerous books that offer help and suggestions on how to change and maintain a gluten-free lifestyle. A quick search on the internet will bring up an endless number of websites that offer tips on cooking, eating out, making your kitchen safe and how to talk to friends and relatives about your new lifestyle.

But Celiacs aren't the only ones who need to change how they live. The friends and relatives of the Celiac also need to change. They need to be conscious of avoiding cross-contamination. They need to be aware of where they put their food, what they touch after eating foods that contain gluten, what products in addition to food contain gluten, and so on. They need to learn to read ingredient lists and how to recognize all the other names for gluten. If the Celiac is a child, they need to learn how to cook with gluten-free ingredients. A quick search on the internet turned up – well – nothing. No tips or tricks for non-Celiacs to help them learn to live with a Celiac. No discussions on the challenges of living with a Celiac. No support groups for non-Celiacs who live with someone who needs to eat gluten-free.

For a Celiac, avoiding gluten is a daily part of life. For the non-Celiac who lives with them, it's ALSO a daily part of life. If you choose to live in a combined household (gluten-free eaters and gluten eaters in the same house), it's different because the non-Celiac can still eat gluten. It might be easier to make the entire household change to gluten-free, but not everyone makes that choice. Many of us choose to live in a combined household.

What is it like for the non-Celiacs? What are their challenges, frustrations and joys? If you are the Celiac, don't believe you are the only one who has to learn to live with a gluten-free lifestyle. The people around you have to learn to live with YOUR gluten-free lifestyle and be conscious of gluten and cross-contamination on a daily basis, too. They have their own difficulties, frustrations and challenges.

Emma's Story

My 4-year old sister, Aivah, has Celiac disease. She was diagnosed when she was 14 months old, so I have been living with someone who follows a gluten-free lifestyle for almost 4 years.

A year and a half ago, my Nana was diagnosed with Celiac disease. Earlier this year, my brother and two more of my sisters were diagnosed with Celiac disease. There are two of us seven siblings who are NOT Celiacs.

I know how difficult and challenging it can be to change to a gluten-free lifestyle and change most of what you're used to eating. It doesn't matter if you're a toddler, a teenager or an adult. It can be scary, frustrating and time-consuming.

There are lots of websites and books that tell people with Celiac disease or a gluten sensitivity how to live a gluten-free lifestyle. But they aren't the only ones that have to learn to live with the challenges of a gluten-free lifestyle. Those of us who can still eat foods that contain gluten, who live in the same house as someone who needs to eat gluten-free, have our own challenges. There are times when it's just not easy. It's frustrating and irritating and time consuming, sometimes.

"Clean the counter!" "Wipe off your mouth before sharing that bottle of pop!" "Don't use my makeup brush!" "Don't leave your gluten food out!" These comments, among others, is what I hear day in and day out at my house. Living with a Celiac is by no means easy, and can be frustrating. And annoying. Frankly, I do a pretty good job cleaning my gluten up and not contaminating the gluten-free items. I know what is and what is not gluten-free. I know how to read labels. I had better, for having to deal with it for 4 years, right?

Yes, it is frustrating for Celiacs, but no one ever thinks about how the non-Celiacs feel. It can be hard to have friends over because I have to remind them about gluten and what foods contain gluten and which ones don't. I have to remind them not to set their gluten foods on counters or tables, and if they do to remind them to wash the counter or table off. I have to remind them not to offer food and/or candy to the little kids unless they ask us first – so we can read the ingredients to make sure it's a safe, gluten-free food.

I constantly need to watch what my gluten foods touch so I don't contaminate the Celiacs. If I'm eating a cookie at the computer and type on the keyboard, I have to wash off the keyboard when I'm done because the gluten that was on my fingers from my cookie is now on the keyboard. I can't share drinking glasses or pop bottles with a Celiac, if I am eating something with gluten in it. My mouth can leave enough gluten on the glass or bottle to make them sick. I fully understand the reason for this and am sometimes overly cautious, but it is something I need to be conscious of all the time. Something as simple as dropping a few gluten crumbs in the wrong place could make one of the Celiacs sick for 2-3 days. When one of them gets sick from cross-contamination (no matter where the gluten contamination came from) I feel bad and wonder if I caused it. My Nana tells us we're only human and accidents happen, so just try to be careful. She gets contaminated more from her own mistakes than from the mistakes of the others in the house.

Gluten is a daily concern for Celiacs, but gluten is also a daily concern for anyone who lives with a Celiac. We "gluten-eaters" have to worry about where the gluten is and cross-contamination and know how to read ingredient lists, too. The only difference is we can still eat foods that have gluten in them.

2 WEEK MENU PLAN

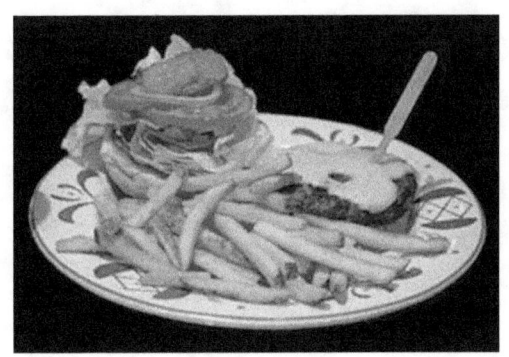

2 Week Menu Plan

Day 1

BREAKFAST
Breakfast Frittata (recipe)
GF Toast with fruit spread
Coffee / Juice

LUNCH
Chicken Salad in Tomato Cup (recipe)
Lays Potato Chips
Milk (or milk alternative)

DINNER
Turkey or beef Tacos (recipe)
GF Refried beans
Beverage of choice

Day 2

BREAKFAST
Kix cereal with milk (or milk alternative)
Juice

LUNCH
GF Hard Salami slices (read ingredients)
GF Crackers or GF toast
Apple slices with GF peanut butter
Milk (or milk alternative)

DINNER
Turkey Wild Rice Casserole (recipe)
Green beans (canned or fresh steamed)
Chocolate milk

Day 3

BREAKFAST
Cream of Rice Cereal (recipe)
Fresh strawberries or blackberries
Juice

LUNCH
GF Turkey on GF toast with lettuce, tomato,
GF mayonnaise
Fritos
Milk (or milk alternative)

DINNER
Pork Chops w/mushroom gravy (recipe)
Baked potato w/butter or sour cream
Carrots (canned or fresh)
Beverage of choice

Day 4

BREAKFAST
Fried Eggs
GF toast w/fruit spread
Fresh Fruit with Honey Glaze (recipe)
Juice

LUNCH
Spinach & Strawberry Salad (recipe)
GF Crackers
Milk, coffee or tea

DINNER
Turkey Chili (recipe)
Easy Cornbread (recipe)
Corn (canned or fresh)
Beverage of choice

Day 5

BREAKFAST
Scrambled Eggs
GF Bacon or sausage
GF Toast w/peanut butter
Juice or milk

LUNCH
Mexican Bean Dip (recipe)
GF Corn tortilla chips
Milk (or milk alternative)

DINNER
Stuffed Mushrooms (recipe)
Creamed potatoes w/fresh parsley
Steamed broccoli
Beverage of choice

Day 6

BREAKFAST
GF cold cereal w/milk (or milk alternative)
Sliced kiwi's and oranges
Juice or milk

LUNCH
Ham sandwich on GF bread w/lettuce & tomato
GF pretzels
Milk or tea

DINNER
Crockpot Beef Roast (recipe)
Beverage of choice

Day 7

BREAKFAST
GF toast w/peanut butter
Frozen Breakfast (recipe)
Coffee, tea or juice

LUNCH
Ham & lettuce wraps (recipe)
GF potato chips
Apple slices
Milk or tea

DINNER
Homemade Chicken Noodle Soup (recipe)
Beverage of choice

Day 8

BREAKFAST
Yogurt Apples (recipe)
GF Rice cakes w/peanut butter
Coffee or juice

LUNCH
Chicken Noodle Soup (leftovers)
GF Crackers
Milk or green tea

DINNER
Hamburgers on GF Buns
GF French Fries
Celery & carrot sticks
Beverage of choice

Day 9

BREAKFAST
Fluffy Pancakes (recipe)
Pure maple syrup or fruit spread
GF bacon or sausage
Pure orange juice

LUNCH
GF Hot dogs on GF buns
GF Tater Tots
Milk

DINNER
Chicken Fajitas (recipe)
Mango Salsa (recipe)
Brown rice or GF refried beans
Beverage of choice

Day 10

BREAKFAST
GF cold cereal w/milk
Banana
Fruit juice

LUNCH
Deviled eggs (recipe)
GF Crackers
GF Corn chips
Milk or juice

DINNER
Vegetable Stir Fry (recipe)
Fried Rice (recipe)
Beverage of choice

Day 11

BREAKFAST
Apple Cakes (recipe)
Fruit spread
Fruit or vegetable juice

LUNCH
Lettuce salad w/tomatoes, cucumbers & dressing
GF rice cake w/peanut butter
Juice or milk

DINNER
Homemade GF Pizza (recipe)
Fresh dinner salad with GF dressing
Beverage of choice

Day 12

BREAKFAST
Cinnamon French toast (recipe)
Scrambled eggs w/cheese (recipe)
Coffee or juice

LUNCH
Grilled hamburger patty
Tomato & cucumber slices
GF Potato chips
Milk or tea

DINNER
Coconut Chicken and Rice (recipe)
Jasmine rice
Beverage of choice

Day 13

BREAKFAST
Fried eggs
GF toast
Vegetable or fruit juice

LUNCH
Peanut butter sandwich on GF bread
Pickles
Milk or tea

DINNER
Crockpot BBQ Ribs (recipe)
Boiled potatoes
Beverage of choice

Day 14

BREAKFAST
Hash Brown Breakfast Pie (recipe)
GF toast
Apple juice

LUNCH
Open Face Rice Cake Sandwiches (recipe)
GF Potato chips
Milk or tea

DINNER
Turkey Burgers & Gravy (recipe)
Mashed Potatoes
Steamed asparagus
Beverage of choice

SNACKS

Soy or coconut milk yogurt
½ cup almonds or cashews
GF Banana Bread (recipe)
GF Pretzels
1 cup grapes (red or green)
Fresh strawberries w/GF chocolate syrup
GF Corn chips
Applesauce
Cantaloupe slices
Cream puffs w/fresh fruit & whipped cream (recipe)
Chocolate filled cream puffs (recipe)
Celery & carrot sticks w/dressing
Apple slices w/peanut butter
Chocolate Mayonnaise Cupcakes (recipe)
Divine GF Coconut Cupcakes (recipe)
Best GF Bread (recipe)

RECIPES

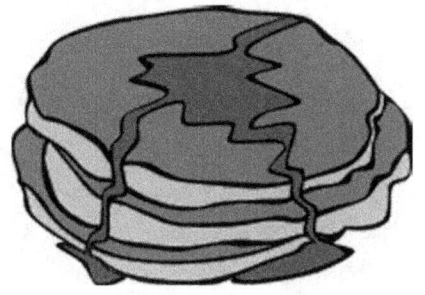

Breakfast Frittata

Serves 4

Ingredients:

½ cup milk or milk alternative
4 eggs
½ cup chopped celery
¼ cup chopped onion
¼ tsp black pepper

2 Tbl GF margarine or butter
1 cup diced potatoes
10-15 fresh spinach leaves
1 tsp GF seasoned salt
½ tsp dried basil

Directions:

In a small bowl combine eggs, milk, basil and pepper. Whip with wire whisk until combined. Set aside.

I large oven-proof frying pan melt margarine (butter) over medium heat. Add potatoes and celery. Sprinkle with seasoned salt and cook over medium heat, stirring occasionally, until potatoes are tender and slightly browned. Add onion and cook 5 minutes until onions are soft and translucent. Lay spinach leaves over top of potato mixture, covering completely. Leave ½ inch of space around edge.

Stir egg mixture to combine, again, and pour over potato mixture in pan. Cook for 5 minutes on medium heat. Remove pan from heat and place under broiling element for 5 – 10 minutes, until top is puffy and slightly browned. Remove from broiler and cut into pie-shaped slices. Serve immediately.

Suggestions:

If you don't have an oven-proof pan, cook on top of the stove until edges are solid and center is slightly liquid. Pour 2-3 Tbl water along edge of mixture. Cover immediately and cook on low heat for 5-10 minutes until steam has cooked top of mixture.

Add one or more of the following:

½ cup cooked chicken, ham or bacon
½ cup broccoli flowerets
¼ cup chopped green chilies

** Add 1 egg for each 1 cup of additional ingredients

Chicken Salad in Tomato Cup

Serves 4

Ingredients:

2 cup diced, cooked chicken
¼ cup chopped onion
1 cup grapes, halved
½ cup mayonnaise
¼ tsp GF dried basil
¼ tsp pepper

½ cup chopped celery
½ cup dried cranberries
¼ cup shredded carrots
4 Tbl milk or milk alternative
1 tsp GF seasoned salt
4 fresh tomatoes

Directions:

In small bowl combine mayonnaise, milk seasoned salt pepper and basil. Stir to combine and set aside.

In large bowl combine remaining ingredients, except tomatoes. Stir to combine. Pour mayonnaise mixture over chicken mixture and stir to coat.

Slice tomatoes into quarters with an "X" almost to bottom of tomato. Be careful not to slice all the way through tomato. Gently pull quartered sections of tomato apart to form "cup".

Place ¼ of chicken salad in center of each tomato.

Turkey or Beef Tacos

Serves 4

Ingredients:

1 lb ground turkey or beef
1 small chopped onion
1 tsp GF dried basil
¼ cup chopped green chilies
½ tsp GF garlic powder

½ cup GF chunky salsa
¼ cup chopped celery
½ tsp seasoned salt
¼ tsp GF ground cumin
8 GF corn tortillas (hard or soft)

Directions:

In large skillet cook ground turkey or beef until almost cooked through. Add onions, celery and spices. Cook, stirring occasionally, until meat is cooked completely. Add salsa and chilies and continue to cook for 5-6 minutes.

Spoon 2-3 Tbl of meat mixture onto center of tortilla. Top with desired toppings.

Suggested Toppings:

Chopped tomatoes
Shredded lettuce
Shredded cheese or dairy-free cheese
Sour cream or Tofu sour cream
Additional chunky salsa
Picante sauce

Turkey Wild Rice Casserole

Serves 4

Ingredients:

½ cup wild rice   ½ cup white rice
2 cup diced, cooked turkey   2 cup GF chicken broth
2- ½ cup water   2/tsp GF cornstarch
3 Tbl chopped onion   ½ cup chopped celery
1 tsp seasoned salt   1 tsp GF dried basil
½ tsp pepper

Directions:

Preheat oven to 350 degrees.

In large bowl mix chicken broth and water. Add cornstarch and stir to dissolve cornstarch. Set aside.

Oil bottom and sides of 2 quart casserole dish. Place diced turkey evenly over bottom of pan. Spread white rice and wild rice evenly over bottom of pan. Sprinkle rice with chopped celery and chopped onion. Sprinkle with basil, salt and pepper. Gently pour chicken broth mixture over ingredients in casserole dish.

Cover casserole dish with tight fitting cover or aluminum foil. Bake 50 – 60 minutes until rice is tender. Remove casserole dish from oven, uncover and stir. Replace cover and let rest for 5 minutes before serving.

Cream of Rice Cereal

Serves 1

Ingredients:

½ cup cream of rice cereal   1 cup water
½ cup milk or milk alternative   2 tsp honey
¼ tsp cinnamon   ¼ tsp GF vanilla

Directions:

Place water and rice cereal in small saucepan. Cook on medium heat, stirring constantly, until mixture starts to thicken (about 5 minutes).

Remove from heat and stir in honey, vanilla and cinnamon. Spoon cereal into bowl and top with milk.

Suggestions:

Add fresh sliced strawberries, blueberries or blackberries to bowl of cereal

Replace honey with 1 tsp granulated sugar

Replace honey with 1 tsp GF brown sugar

Replace honey with 1 tsp pure maple syrup

Pork Chops with Mushroom Gravy

Serves 4

Ingredients

4 bone-in pork chops
1 small onion, thinly sliced
1 tsp seasoned salt
¼ tsp GF black pepper
1 cup GF vegetable broth
¼ cup water

1 cup sliced mushrooms
¼ cup chopped celery
½ tsp GF dried basil
2 Tbl vegetable oil
2 tsp cornstarch

Heat oil in large skillet. While skillet is heating, coat both sides of each pork chop with salt, pepper and basil.

When pan is hot, place pork chops in pan and cook until bottom is browned. Depending on thickness of pork chops, this should take about 5 – 10 minutes.

Turn pork chops over in pan so cooked side is facing up. Add onions and celery to pan. Cover and cook an additional 5 – 10 minutes until bottoms of pork chops are browned. Remove pork chops from pan.

Add mushrooms to pan and cook until tender. Stir occasionally to combine with onions and celery. Add ½ cup vegetable broth to hot pan, stirring and scraping with wooden spoon to loosen browned pieces on bottom of pan. Add remaining broth and water/cornstarch mixture. Stir until gravy thickens. Return pork chops to pan and cover with mushroom gravy. Cover and heat for 5 minutes until pork chops are heated through.

Serve immediately.

Fresh Fruit with Honey Glaze

Serves 2

Ingredients:

1 cup fresh strawberries
½ cup fresh raspberries
½ cup fresh blackberries
1 banana. Sliced
½ cup fresh blueberries
¼ cup honey
½ tsp GF vanilla

Directions:

Slice strawberries into quarters. Place all fresh fruits in large bowl.

In small bowl, combine honey and vanilla. Stir with wire whisk to combine. Pour honey mixture over fresh fruit. Stir gently to coat all fruit with honey mixture. Serve immediately.

Suggestions:

Add or replace with any of the following fruits:

       Sliced peaches
       Slices nectarines
       Pineapple chunks
       Sliced apple
       Sliced mango
       Sliced papaya

Spinach & Strawberry Salad

Serves 4

Ingredients:

4 cups fresh baby spinach leaves
1 cup sliced strawberries
½ c chopped walnuts or pecans

Strawberry Vinaigrette:

1 pint fresh strawberries
¼ C apple cider vinegar
¾ tsp GF dried basil
¼ tsp GF thyme
½ tsp salt
¼ tsp black pepper
½ tsp granulated sugar
¼ olive oil or vegetable oil

In large bowl, combine spinach, strawberry slices and nuts. Gently toss to combine. Set aside.

Puree strawberries in blender or food processor. Place pureed berries in large bowl. Add vinegar and spices and blend with wire whisk. While whisking, pour thin steady stream of oil into mixture and whisk until thoroughly combined.

Pour desired amount of strawberry vinaigrette over salad. (Remaining vinaigrette can be stored in refrigerator for 2 -3 days. Mix again before serving.) Gently toss to coat spinach and strawberries with vinaigrette.

Serve immediately.

Turkey Chili

Serves 4

Ingredients:

1 lb ground turkey
¼ cup chopped onion
2 Tbl vegetable oil
1 – 15 oz can kidney beans, not drained
1 – 16 oz can tomato sauce
¼ cup chopped celery
¼ cup chopped green pepper
1 large garlic clove, finely chopped
1 tsp seasoned salt
½ - 1 tsp GF chili powder (to taste)

Directions:

In large skillet, brown ground turkey in oil. Add onion, celery, green pepper and garlic. Cook for 10 minutes, until onions and peppers are tender.

In large kettle, combine tomato sauce, kidney beans, salt and chili powder. Stir to combine. Add cooked turkey mixture to sauce. Cook covered for 20 – 25 minutes.

Serve in individual bowls topped with shredded cheese and sour cream (or dairy-free cheese alternative and tofu sour cream).

Easy Gluten-free Cornbread

Serves 4

Ingredients:

½ cup rice flour
½ cup tapioca flour
¼ cup cornstarch
¾ cup GF cornmeal
½ tsp xanthan gum
¼ cup granulated sugar
2 tsp GF baking powder
1 cup milk (or milk alternative)
¼ cup vegetable oil
1 egg

Directions:

Preheat oven to 400 degrees. Oil 8" square pan.

In medium bowl combine dry ingredients. Stir to combine. Add milk, egg and oil and mix until dry ingredients are moistened. Do not over mix.

Pour batter into prepared pan. Bake 20 – 25 minutes or until golden brown and toothpick inserted in center comes out clean.

Serve warm with honey.

Mexican Bean Dip

Serves 4

Ingredients:

1 – 15 oz. can GF black beans
1 – 15 oz. can GF refried beans
¼ cup chopped onion
1 cup shredded lettuce
¼ cup sour cream(Tofu sour cream)
½ cup shredded cheese or cheese alternative

¼ cup chopped green chilies
¼ cup chunky salsa
3 Roma tomatoes, chopped
½ tsp GF garlic powder
GF corn tortilla chips
½ tsp GF cumin

Directions:

In large saucepan combine black beans, refried beans, salsa, onion, garlic powder, cumin and green chilies. Heat over medium heat, stirring occasionally, until heated through. Continue to cook 5-10 minutes for flavors to combine.

Spoon bean mixture into large bowl. Spread sour cream over top of bean mixture. Sprinkle with lettuce and tomatoes. Add additional cheese if desired.

Serve with GF corn tortilla chips.

Stuffed Mushrooms

Serves 4 – 6

Ingredients:

1-½ lb medium sized mushrooms
½ lb ground pork or turkey
2 Tbl vegetable oil
½ shredded mozzarella cheese (or cheese alternative)
¼ cup GF dry bread crumbs
¼ cup finely chopped onion
¼ tsp GF garlic powder
½ tsp GF dried basil
½ tsp salt
¼ tsp black pepper

Directions:

Preheat oven to 350 degrees.

Remove mushroom stems and finely chop. Heat oil in large skillet over medium heat. Add ground meat, onion, mushroom stems, garlic and spices. Cook 15 minutes until meat is no longer pink, stirring occasionally.

Remove from heat and stir in cheese and bread crumbs. Stir to combine mixture.

Place mushroom caps with rounded side down on parchment-lined cookie sheet. Fill mushroom caps with 2 Tbl of meat mixture. Gently press mixture onto mushroom caps.

Bake for 15 minutes. Remove from oven and serve immediately.

Crockpot Beef Roast

Serves 4

Ingredients:

2 – 3 lb beef roast (chuck roast works well in a crockpot)

4 large potatoes	4 large carrots, peeled
1 small onion	1 bay leaf
2 cloves garlic	½ tsp dried basil
½ tsp salt	black pepper to taste
¼ tsp GF dried rosemary	¼ tsp GF dried thyme
½ cup GF beef stock or broth	

Directions:

Place roast in crockpot. Cut potatoes, onion and carrots into quarters and place on top of roast. Sprinkle ingredients in crockpot with spices and add bay leaf. Pour beef broth into crockpot. Cover and cook on low 6 – 8 hours. Roast can be prepared in 4-5 hours with crockpot on medium.

Frozen Breakfast

Serves 4

Ingredients:

1-15 oz can crushed pineapple
4 bananas, sliced
1 15 oz can peaches in juice
2-10oz pkg frozen strawberries with juice
3 Tbl granulated sugar or honey

Directions:

Drain pineapple and reserve juice for other recipes. Drain peaches and reserve juice for this recipe.

In large bowl combine pineapple, banana slices, peach slices and strawberries with juice.

In small saucepan combine peach juice and sugar or honey. Bring to a boil over medium heat, stirring occasionally. Reduce heat to medium-low and continue to cook 10 – 15 minutes, until liquid has been reduced.

Pour hot peach juice over fruits in bowl. Stir gently to combine.

Spoon fruit and juice into cupcake pans that have been lined with paper liners. Place in freezer for 2 hours or overnight.

Allow fruit cups to sit at room temperatures for 10 minutes before serving. Serve in paper cups or invert onto plate and remove cupcake paper.

Ham and Turkey Lettuce Wraps

Serves 4

Ingredients:

8 pieces of thin sliced deli ham
8 pieces of thin sliced deli turkey
16 large Romaine lettuce leaves
4 dill or sweet pickles, halved
8 thin tomato slices
Mayonnaise

Directions:

Break off hard bottoms of lettuce leaves, so the height of lettuce leaf is slightly taller than the width of the ham/turkey slices.

Lay lettuce leaf on flat surface. Spread a thin layer of mayonnaise on lettuce leaf. Place 1 slice of ham and 1 slice of turkey in center of lettuce leaf. Top with 1 tomato slice. Place 1 pickle half near outer edge of lettuce leaf. Fold edge of lettuce leaf over pickle. Roll lettuce and meat around pickle half. Secure with toothpick.

Dipping Sauces:

Western dressing
Ranch dressing
Italian dressing

Homemade Chicken Soup
with Gluten-free Noodles

Serves 8

Ingredients:

1 whole chicken	1 cup diced celery
½ cup diced onion	1 – ½ cup diced carrots
2 small cloves garlic	2 Tbl GF seasoned salt
1 tsp salt	½ tsp black pepper
1 bay leaf	2 Tbl GF dried parsley
1 tsp GF dried basil	4 cups water
2 cups GF vegetable broth	4 cups GF chicken broth

Directions:

Rinse chicken inside and out and place in 6 quart kettle. Bring to a boil over medium high heat. Reduce heat to medium, cover and cook for 2 hours.

Remove from heat and take chicken from kettle. Remove skin and bones from chicken. Cut half the chicken into bite sized pieces and return to kettle. Refrigerate remaining half of chicken for future recipes. Cook soup on medium low heat while you prepare the GF noodles. (This reduces the liquid and enhances the flavor of the soup.

Gluten-free Noodles

½ cup tapioca flour	3 Tbl potato starch flour
½ cup cornstarch	½ tsp salt
1 Tbl xanthan gum	2 large eggs
1 Tbl vegetable oil	

Combine dry ingredients in medium bowl and set aside. In small bowl, whisk together eggs and oil. Pour egg mixture into flour mixture and mi with a fork to combine. Dough will be thick and stiff.

Dust bread board or counter with tapioca flour. Knead dough until dough Is firm and no longer sticky, adding more tapioca flour if needed. Cut dough into quarters. Roll first quarter of dough to 1/8" thickness. Slice into strips of desired width. Gently place cut noodles into a large saucepan of boiling water to which 1 Tbl of oil has been added. Cook 3 – 5 minutes. Remove noodles with slotted spoon and add to soup kettle. Roll, slice and boil remaining noodles and add to soup. Heat for 10 minutes and serve.

Yogurt Apples

Serves 4

Ingredients:

4 apples, sliced and cored
4 Tbl honey
1/2 C chopped almonds
1 container GF yogurt (vanilla or flavored)

Directions:

Pour yogurt into 4 small bowls. Place apple slices on small microwave safe plate. Microwave 2 – 3 minutes. Remove from microwave and drizzle warm apples with honey. Place apples on top of yogurt. Sprinkle with chopped almonds.

Serve and enjoy.

Fluffy Pancakes

Serves 4

Ingredients:

¼ cup rice flour
½ cup tapioca flour
¼ cup potato starch flour
1 tsp xanthan gun
1 tsp baking powder
2 tsp GF vanilla
2 eggs
2 Tbl vegetable oil
1 cup milk (or milk alternative)
1 tsp cinnamon

Directions:

Heat oil on griddle or large skillet over medium heat. In medium bowl combine flours and xanthan gum. Mix with wire whisk to incorporate xanthan gum. Add remaining ingredients. Mix with wire whisk until blended.

Pour ¼ cup of batter onto hot griddle. Cook for 3 minutes or until bubbles begin to form on top of batter. Flip pancake over and cook another 3 minutes.

Serving Suggestions:

Serve with pure maple syrup

Serve with fresh blackberries or strawberries

Add ½ cup chocolate chips to batter before cooking.

Add ½ cup fresh blueberries to batter before cooking.

Spread pancake with peanut butter and jelly and roll up for fun "finger food"

Chicken Fajitas with Mango Salsa

Serves 4

Ingredients:

2 Tbl vegetable oil
1 red pepper, thin strips
1 large onion, sliced thin
¼ cup GF chicken broth
¼ tsp salt
½ tsp GF dried basil
½ C diced tomatoes
½ C tofu sour cream
2 boneless, skinless chicken breasts

1 green pepper, thin strips
1 yellow pepper, thin strips
1 large garlic clove, finely chopped
1 Tbl GF seasoned salt
¼ tsp pepper
½ C GF chunky salsa
½ C shredded cheese (or non-dairy cheese)
4-6 GF tortillas

Directions:

Cut chicken breasts into thin strips. In small bowl combine seasoned salt, salt, basil and pepper. Sprinkle mixture on chicken strips, coating all sides.

Heat oil in large skillet or wok on medium high heat. When oil is hot, add chicken strips and cook 5 – 6 minutes until completely cooked and no longer pink.

Add onions, garlic and pepper strips. Cook 10 minutes until peppers are tender and onions are soft. Add chicken broth and salsa. Cook 10 minutes until heated through.

Serve on gluten-free tortillas with dice tomatoes, cheese (or non-dairy cheese alternative), sour cream (or tofu sour cream). Top with Mango Salsa.

Quick and Easy Mango Salsa

Serves 4

Ingredients:

1 mango (peeled & chopped)
1/2 fresh pineapple (peeled & chopped)
    (you can use 1 small can of pineapple chunks or crushed pineapple)
6-7 strawberries (chopped)
2 Roma tomatoes (chopped)
1 small onion (chopped – about 1/4 cup)
1/2 red pepper (chopped)
1/2 green pepper (chopped)
1/2 yellow pepper (chopped)
3/4 C chunky salsa (we use Pace mild chunky salsa to hold it all together and add a little spice)
1/2 tsp ground cumin

Stir all ingredients together in medium sized bowl. Eat. (That's how "Quick & Easy" it is.)

If you don't have all the ingredients (such as strawberries or colored peppers, change it up a little for an entirely different flavor. Maybe add chopped peaches, or chopped apples . . . get creative!)

This salsa is also very tasty served as a dip with gluten-free corn tortilla chips.

Deviled Eggs

Serves 4

Ingredients:

8 hardboiled eggs
½ cup GF mayonnaise
2 Tbl seasoned salt
2 Tbl finely chopped onion
½ tsp salt
¼ tsp black pepper
1 Tbl yellow mustard
¼ tsp GF dried basil
GF paprika for decoration

Directions:

Cut eggs in half lengthwise. Gently remove yolks, being careful not to break whites. Set aside.

In medium bowl mash egg yolks with fork. Add onion and seasonings to egg yolks, stirring to combine. Add mayonnaise and mustard, mixing until smooth.

Spoon egg yolk mixture into egg white halves. Sprinkle with paprika.

Suggestion:

You can fill a zip lock lunch bag with the egg yolk mixture. Zip top shut and cut off corner of bag ½" across. Pipe filling into egg white halves. Sprinkle with paprika.

Vegetable Stir Fry

Serves 4

Ingredients:

½ cup diced celery
1 cup julienne carrots
½ cup sliced onion
½ cup green pepper strips
½ cup red pepper strips
1 cup broccoli florets
1 cup pea pods
1 cup diced bok choy (optional)
½ cup chicken broth
1 Tbl cornstarch
1 clove garlic, finely chopped
3 Tbl vegetable oil
2 Tsp GF tamari or GF soy sauce

Directions:

Heat oil in large skillet or wok, over medium heat. When oil is hot, add carrots, celery and pea pods. Cook 5 minutes. Add onions, broccoli, peppers, bok choy and garlic. Cook an additional 10 minutes.

While vegetables are cooking, in small bowl combine chicken broth, soy sauce and cornstarch. Stir until cornstarch is dissolved. Pour mixture over vegetables in pan, stirring until sauce thickens.

Serve over hot rice or GF spaghetti noodles.

Apple Cakes

Serves 4

Ingredients:

1 ripe banana
2 Tbl vegetable oil
1 cup milk (or alternative milk)
½ cup sorghum flour
1 tsp xanthan gum
½ tsp salt
2 tsp cinnamon

2 eggs
2 Tbl pure maple syrup
1 cup tapioca flour
½ cup potato starch flour
1 Tbl GF baking powder
2 C peeled, grated apple
¼ tsp nutmeg

Directions:

In large bowl mix banana and eggs with electric mixer. Add oil and soy milk. Mix until well blended.

In medium bowl combine flours, baking powder, salt, cinnamon and nutmeg. Add to banana mixture. Mix well with fork.

Stir in apples. Stir until apples are well incorporated.

Heat oil on griddle or large skillet. Drop spoonsful onto hot pan forming circle about 3" across. (An ice cream scoop works great for this.)

Heat cakes over medium heat until bubbles appear. Flip cake and cook second side until cooked through and brown around the edges.

Serve with maple syrup or fruit spread.

GF Pizza

Serves 4

Ingredients:

1 cup brown rice flour	1 cup tapioca flour
1 cup cornstarch	1 ½ tsp xanthan gum
2 tsp granulated sugar	¾ tsp salt
1 package dry yeast	1 – 1 ½ cup warm water, divided
2 eggs	3 Tbl vegetable oil

1 tsp apple cider vinegar (optional)
GF Pizza sauce   Desired toppings
1 cup shredded mozzarella cheese (or cheese alternative)

Directions:

Preheat oven to 400 degrees. Line large pizza pan or large cookie sheet with parchment paper.

In small bowl, combine dry yeast, sugar and ½ cup warm water. Set aside until bubbles foam on top surface.

In large bowl combine flours, salt and xanthan gum. Add 1 cup warm water, eggs, oil and vinegar. Mix on low until combined. Add yeast mixture and beat for 5 minutes until dough is smooth, but not runny. (Add more rice flour if needed.)

Spoon dough onto prepared pan. Oil hands and smooth crust to edges of pan.

Prebake crust for 10 minutes, until slightly browned. Remove from oven and top with sauce and desired toppings.

Return to oven and bake 15 – 20 mi8nutes until cheese is melted and crust is browned.

Cinnamon French Toast

Serves 2

Ingredients:

4 slices GF bread
2 eggs
½ cup milk (or milk alternative)
½ tsp GF cinnamon
1 tsp granulated sugar
2 Tbl GF margarine (or butter)

Directions:

In medium bowl, combine eggs, milk, cinnamon and sugar. Mix with wire whisk until well combined.

Heat small skillet on medium heat. Add margarine (butter) and stir until bottom of pan is coated.

Place 1 slice of bread in egg mixture, coating both sides of bread. Place coated bread in hot skillet. Cook 2 – 3 minutes until bottom is browned. Turn bread over and cook second side for 2 – 3 minutes. Remove to oven-safe plate and keep warm in oven (200 degrees).

Cook additional slices of bread.

Suggested Toppings:

Serve with pure maple syrup

Serve with GF applesauce

Serve with peanut butter or almond butter

Coconut Chicken and Rice

Serves 4

Ingredients:

2 boneless, skinless chicken breasts
1 – 13.5 oz can coconut milk   ½ tsp GF seasoned salt
¼ tsp GF red chili paste   ¼ cup chopped onion
1 clove garlic, finely chopped   2 Tbl vegetable oil
4 C cooked Basmati rice

Directions:

Cut chicken into 1" pieces. Sprinkle with seasoned salt. Place oil in large, deep skillet and heat on medium heat. When pan is hot, add chicken pieces to pan. Cook chicken 10 – 12 minutes until cooked completely.

Add onions and garlic. Cook for 4-5 minutes until onions are translucent, stirring occasionally.

Pour coconut milk over chicken mixture. Add chili paste to mixture and stir until combined. Continue to cook over medium heat 10 – 15 minutes, until coconut milk has thickened and reduced.

Serve over hot cooked rice.

Crockpot BBQ Ribs

Serves 4

Ingredients:

8 beef or pork ribs
1 – 16 oz bottle of GF BBQ sauce
¼ cup chopped onions
¼ cup chopped celery
¼ cup shredded carrots
¼ cup chopped green pepper
¼ cup chopped red pepper
1 tsp GF dried basil
1 cup water

Directions:

In small bowl combine BBQ sauce, water and basil. Stir to combine and set aside.

Place ribs in crockpot. Place onion, celery, carrots and peppers over ribs. Pour BBQ sauce mixture over ribs, making sure to coat all ribs.

Cover crockpot and cook on low 6 – 8 hours until tender. (Can be cooked on medium 3 – 4 hours.)

Hash Brown Breakfast Pie

Serves 4

Ingredients:

3 cup GF frozen hash browns
1 cup diced cooked ham
½ cup chopped broccoli
3 large eggs
1 tsp GF seasoned salt

3 Tbl GF margarine, melted
1 cup shredded mozzarella cheese
 (or dairy-free cheese alternative)
½ cup milk (or dairy-free milk)
¼ tsp black pepper

Directions:

Oil bottom and sides of 9" pie pan. Preheat oven to 350 degrees.

Thaw frozen hash browns between layers of paper towel, to remove excess moisture. Press potatoes into bottom of pie pan.

Drizzle melted margarine over potatoes. Bake for 10 - 15 minutes, until lightly browned. Remove from oven and cool while you prepare the remaining ingredients.

In medium bowl combine ham, cheese and broccoli. Spoon into potato crust.

In small bowl combine eggs, milk, salt and pepper. Whisk until well blended. Pour egg mixture over ham, cheese and broccoli.

Bake for 20 – 25 minutes or until eggs are set. Let stand for 5 minutes before serving. Cut into pie-shaped wedges to serve.

Open Face Rice Cake Sandwiches

Serves 4

Ingredients

8 GF plain rice cakes
8 slices deli honey ham
8 tomato slices
Shredded lettuce
8 slices American cheese (or cheese alternative)
Mayonnaise or Thousand Island salad dressing

Directions:

Spread mayonnaise or Thousand Island dressing on each rice cake. Top with shredded cheese and tomato slice. Place 1 slice deli ham on top of tomato. Top ham with cheese slice.

Place topped rice cakes on parchment lined cookie sheet. Place pan under broiler for 1 minute, until cheese is melted.

Serve and enjoy!

Turkey Burgers & Gravy

Serves 4

Ingredients:

1 lb ground turkey
½ cup chopped celery
½ cup shredded carrots
2 Tbl GF dried parsley
½ tsp salt
1 egg

½ cup chopped mushrooms
¼ cup chopped onions
½ cup GF vegetable protein flakes
¼ tsp black pepper
½ tsp GF paprika

½ cup water
4 Tbl cornstarch

¾ cup GF chicken broth
3 Tbl vegetable oil

Directions:

In small bowl combine water and cornstarch. Stir until cornstarch is dissolved and set aside.

In large bowl combine remaining ingredients EXCEPT oil and chicken broth. Mix until evenly combined. Form into 8 patties.

Heat oil in large skillet on medium heat. Place patties in pan and cook 8 – 10 minutes, until bottoms are browned. Flip patties over and cook and additional 8 – 10 minutes. Remove patties from pan and set aside.

Add chicken broth to hot pan, stirring to loosen cooked meat pieces from bottom of pan. Reduce heat to low. Add water/cornstarch mixture and stir constantly until mixture thickens. Place turkey patties into gravy and spoon gravy over each patty. Cover and cook on low heat for additional 5 minutes.

Snack Recipes

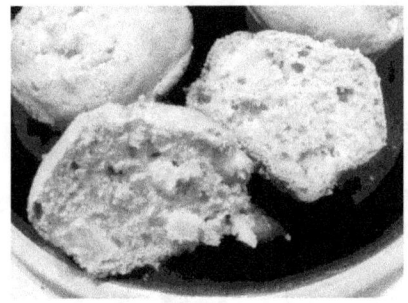

Banana Nut Bread

Makes 1 loaf

Ingredients:

1 cup brown rice flour
1 cup white rice flour
¼ cup corn starch
¼ cup tapioca flour
1 tsp xanthan gum
1 Tbl GF baking powder
½ tsp salt
1 egg
½ cup GF margarine
2/3 cup honey or brown sugar
3 large bananas, mashed
½ cup walnuts or pecans

Directions:

Preheat oven to 350 degrees. Grease one 9 4 loaf pan and dust with granulated sugar.

In large bowl combine flours, xanthan gum, baking powder and salt. Set aside.

In medium bowl, mix bananas, margarine, egg and honey (or brown sugar) on medium speed until combined. Stir in nuts.

Add wet ingredients to dry ingredients and stir until thoroughly combined. Spoon batter into pan, smoothing top. Bake for 40 – 45 minutes or until top starts to crack and knife inserted into center comes out clean.

Cream Puffs

Makes 12 cream puffs

Ingredients:

1 cup water
½ cup margarine
1/3 cup potato starch flour
1/3 cup rice flour
1/3 cup tapioca flour
½ tsp salt
1 Tbl granulated sugar
4 eggs

Directions:

Preheat oven to 400 degrees. Line cookie sheet with parchment paper.

In medium saucepan combine water and margarine. Bring to rapid boil over medium-high heat. Once mixture boils, remove from heat.

In medium bowl combine flours, salt and sugar. Pour dry mixture into liquid mixture in saucepan all at once. Stir vigorously with wooden spoon until mixture forms a ball that leaves sides of pan.

Add eggs, one at a time, beating well with wooden spoon (or hand held mixer) after each addition.

Drop 12 spoonsful onto prepared cookie sheet. Bake at 400 for 15 minutes. Reduce heat to 350 degrees and bake an additional 30 – 35 minutes until browned.

Remove puffs from oven and prick each one with a knife, to allow steam to escape.

Allow to cool before serving. Serve filled fresh fruit, whipped topping, dairy-free whipped topping or chocolate pudding.

Chocolate Mayonnaise Cupcakes

Makes 18 cupcakes

Ingredients:

1 cup rice flour
½ cup tapioca flour
½ cup cornstarch
1-½ tsp xanthan gum
2/3 cup unsweetened cocoa
2/3 cup granulated sugar
1-½ tsp GF baking soda
1 tsp GF baking powder
1 cup GF mayonnaise
2/3 cup water
3 eggs
¼ cup oil

Directions:

Preheat oven to 350 degrees. Line cupcake pan with cupcake papers.

In large bowl combine eggs and sugar. Beat on high for 2 minutes until light and fluffy and pale yellow. Reduce speed to low and blend in mayonnaise and oil.

Add water and mix on low until blended. Add flours, cornstarch and cocoa and mix on low until blended. Add baking powder, baking soda and xanthan gum. Mix on medium speed until mixture thickens.

Fill cupcake papers 2/3 full. Bake for 20 - 25 minutes or until top springs back when pressed lightly.

Cool and frost.

Divine Coconut Cupcakes

Makes 18 cupcakes

Ingredients:

2 13 – 14 oz cans unsweetened coconut milk
1/2 cup tapioca flour
2-1/2 tsp baking powder
3/4 cup margarine (or butter)
1-1/3 cup granulated sugar
1 cup reduced coconut milk (see below)

1 cup rice flour
1/2 cup corn starch
3 large eggs
1 tsp GF vanilla
1-1/2 tsp xanthan gum

Reduced coconut milk:

Pour both cans of coconut milk into deep saucepan. Coconut milk should only fill the pan half way. Heat coconut milk on medium high heat until it boils. (Coconut milk will boil up high in pan, which is why you need a deep saucepan.) Reduce heat to low and gently boil until it is reduced to 1 – 1/2 cups – about 25 – 35 minutes. Stir occasionally so it doesn't burn on the bottom of the pan. Once reduced, the coconut milk with be thick and creamy. Place in refrigerator and cool completely. (You can reduce the coconut milk days ahead and store in the refrigerator until you are ready to bake.)

Cupcakes:

Preheat oven to 350 degrees. In large mixing bowl, combine margarine (or butter) and granulated sugar. Beat on high until smooth and light yellow. Add eggs and beat on high until well blended, about 2 minutes. Turn off mixer, scrape down sides and add rice flour and tapioca flour. Mix on low until well blended. Add 1 cup reduced coconut milk (reserve remaining 1/2 cup for frosting) and vanilla and mix on low until blended. Add cornstarch, baking powder and baking soda and mix until blended.

Line muffin cups with paper cupcake liners. Fill each until 3/4 full. Bake at 350 degrees for 20 – 30 minutes until slightly brown. Top should spring back when pressed lightly. Remove from pans and cool completely before frosting. (Warm cupcakes will melt your frosting.)

(Coconut frosting follows)

Coconut Frosting:

1 cup margarine (or butter)
2-1/2 cup powdered sugar
1/3 cup reduced coconut milk
1/2 tsp GF vanilla

In large mixing bowl, beat margarine until soft and smooth. Add 1 cup of powdered sugar and mix on low until combined. Scrape sides of bowl and add 1 additional cup of powdered sugar. Mix until blended. Add reduced coconut milk and vanilla and mix until well blended. Scrape sides of bowl and add remaining 1/2 cup powdered sugar. Mix until blended. Frost cupcakes with 2 tsp frosting for each cupcake. Sprinkle top of cupcake with sweetened flaked coconut. (If frosting is too thin add a little more powdered sugar or refrigerate before using. Frosting will become firmer if cold. If your kitchen is too hot, the frosting won't set up well.)

Best Gluten-free Bread

Makes 1 loaf

Ingredients:

1-1/3 cup warm water
1 pkg dry yeast
1 Tbl granulated sugar

¼ cup vegetable oil
¼ cup honey
3 eggs
1 tsp salt
1 cup rice flour
1 cup tapioca flour
1 ¼ cup cornstarch
1 ½ tsp xanthan gum
¼ cup ground golden flax seeds

Directions:

Preheat oven to 350 degrees. Grease a 9 x 5 loaf pan. (You can coat the pan with rice flour if desired. If you have a non-stick loaf pan this isn't necessary.)

In large mixing bowl combine water, yeast and sugar. Stir to combine. Set aside until mixture foams on top.

Add eggs, oil and honey to yeast mixture and mix until well blended. Add flours, cornstarch and ground flax seeds and mix on medium until well blended. Scrape down sides of bowl and add xanthan gum. Mix on medium until well blended and dough thickens.

Bake bread for 55 to 60 minutes until crust is golden brown.

Bread is done when crust is golden brown and tapping on the crust give a hollow sound.

*** IMPORTANT STEP TO SUCCESSFUL GLUTEN-FREE BREAD ***
The drastic temperature change from a hot oven to a cold kitchen can cause gluten-free bread to sink in the middle.

When bread is done, turn oven off and leave door open slightly. Leave bread in cooling oven for 15 – 20 minutes. Take bread out of oven and remove from pan. Allow to cool completely before wrapping in plastic wrap. Store in refrigerator.

Bibliography

Lieberman, Shari. The Gluten Connection: How Gluten Sensitivity May Be Sabotaging Your Health-- and What You Can Do to Take Control Now. [Emmaus, Penn.]: Rodale, 2007. Print.

Korn, Danna. Living Gluten-free for Dummies. Hoboken, NJ: Wiley Pub., 2006. Print.

Korn, Danna, and Alessio Fasano. Living Gluten-free for Dummies. Hoboken, NJ: Wiley, 2010. Print.

Petersen, Vikki, and Richard Petersen. The Gluten Effect: How "innocent" Wheat Is Ruining Your Health. [Sunnyvale, CA?]: True Health Pub., 2009. Print

Green, Peter H. R., and Rory Jones. Celiac Disease: a Hidden Epidemic. New York, NY: William Morrow, 2010. Print.

Kids with Celiac Disease : A Family Guide to Raising Happy, Healthy, Gluten-Free Children: Woodbine House, 2001, Print

Fellstone, Diane S. Gluten: Properties, Modifications and Dietary Intolerance. New York: Nova Science, 2011. Print.

Green, Peter H. R., and Rory Jones. Celiac Disease: a Hidden Epidemic. New York: Collins, 2006. Print.

Haas, Sidney V., and Merrill Patterson Haas. Management of Celiac Disease,. Philadelphia: Lippincott, 1951. Print.

Gershwin, M. Eric, and Yehuda Shoenfeld. Autoimmunity, Basic Principles and New Diagnostic Tools. Boston, MA: Published by Blackwell Pub. on Behalf of the New York Academy of Sciences, 2007. Print.

Niewinski, M. "Advances in Celiac Disease and Gluten-Free Diet." Journal of the American Dietetic Association 108.4 (2008): 661-72. Print.

Green, Peter H.R., and Bana Jabri. "Celiac Disease." Annual Review of Medicine 57.1 (2006): 207-21. Print.

Elder, Jennifer Harrison, Meena Shankar, Jonathan Shuster, Douglas Theriaque, Sylvia Burns, and Lindsay Sherrill. "The Gluten-Free, Casein-Free Diet In Autism: Results of A Preliminary Double Blind Clinical Trial." Journal of Autism and Developmental Disorders 36.3 (2006): 413-20. Print.

Libonati, Cleo J. Recognizing Celiac Disease: Signs, Symptoms, Associated Disorders & Complications. Fort Washington, PA: Gluten Free Works Pub., 2007. Print.

Wangen, Stephen. Healthier without Wheat: a New Understanding of Wheat Allergies, Celiac Disease, and Non-celiac Gluten Intolerance. Seattle, WA: Innate Health Pub., 2009. Print.

Braly, James, and Ron Hoggan. Dangerous Grains: Why Gluten Cereal Grains May Be Hazardous to Your Health. New York: Avery, 2002. Print.

Wheat Allergy and Intolerance Information on Wheat-free.org." Wheat-free.org - Wheat Free Recipes, Places to Eat, Suppliers of Ingredients. Web. 17 Feb. 2010. <http://www.wheat-free.org/wheat-allergy.html>.

Celiac Disease - National Digestive Diseases Information Clearinghouse." Home - National Digestive Diseases Information Clearinghouse. Web. 2 May 2010. <http://digestive.niddk.nih.gov/ddiseases/pubs/celiac/>.

Adams, Jefferson. "A Systematic Review of Diagnostic Testing for Celiac Disease Among Patients With Abdominal Symptoms - Celiac.com." Celiac Disease & Gluten-free Diet Information at Celiac.com. 03 June 2010. Web. 24 Nov. 2011. <http://www.celiac.com/articles/22151/1/A-Systematic-Review-of-Diagnostic-Testing-for-Celiac-Disease-Among-Patients-With-Abdominal-Symptoms-/Page1.html>.

"Vaccines: HOME Page for Vaccines and Immunizations Site." Centers for Disease Control and Prevention. Web. 2 Nov. 2011. <http://www.cdc.gov/vaccines>.

National Vaccine Information Center – Vaccine Watch Dog. Web. 14 Oct. 2011. <http://www.nvic.org>.

WAVE - World Association for Vaccine Education. Web. 2 Sept. 2011. <http://www.novaccine.com>.

Celiac Teen. Web. 24 Nov. 2011. <http://www.celiacteen.com>.

Celiac Disease | The University of Chicago Celiac Disease Center. Web. 6 Oct. 2011. <http://www.cureceliacdisease.org>.

Center for Celiac Disease Research: University of Maryland School of Medicine. Web. 17 May. 2011. <http://celiaccenter.org/>.

Adams, Jefferson. "Environmental and Other Factors Can Impair Celiac Disease Diagnosis in Symptomatic Children." 29 June 2010. Web.

Turbin, Tina. "Probiotics: A Future Answer to Celiac Disease?" 13 June 2010. Web.

Stone, Destiny. "Celiac Disease." 26 Mar. 2010. Web. 24 Nov. 2010. <http://www.ncbi.nlm.nih.gov/pmc/articles/PMC2830645/>.

Index

www.ingramcontent.com/pod-product-compliance
Lightning Source LLC
Chambersburg PA
CBHW060244290526
45789CB00001B/182